Physical Education: AN OVERVIEW

SECOND EDITION

BEVERLY L. SEIDEL
Kent State University

MATTHEW C. RESICK
formerly Kent State University

ADDISON-WESLEY PUBLISHING COMPANY

Reading, Massachusetts
Menlo Park, California
London · Amsterdam
Don Mills, Ontario
Sydney

This book is in the

ADDISON-WESLEY SERIES IN PHYSICAL EDUCATION

The photographs on the part and chapter opening pages, unless otherwise indicated, were supplied by the Kent State Department of Physical Education and the authors.

ISBN 0-201-06988-1
ABCDEFGHIJ-MA-798

To Ike
and
To Our Families

Preface

The purposes of this book are: to aid intelligent, well-informed students, today's typical college freshmen, to gain an insight into the broad discipline of physical education; to acquaint students, generally, with the organized body of knowledge embraced within the discipline of physical education; and to show the proper relationship of physical education to the fields of health education and recreation.

The first edition of this book has been criticized by some for its brevity. From years of experience in teaching an introductory course in physical education, the authors are convinced that the textbook for such a course should be characterized by brevity, reference to current research studies, and appeal to the inquiring human nature. We hope this book meets all these criteria. All areas of the field of physical education typically examined in a beginning course are briefly covered; numerous examples of current research are cited; and questions are purposefully left unanswered so that students, given teacher encouragement and guidance, will be motivated by curiosity to undertake further individual and/or group study. No introductory book can do justice to the areas of specialization included in the discipline; therefore, it is our hope that the generalized information contained herein will serve to whet the scholarly appetites of students to seek additional, in-depth knowledge. How can one truly understand a particular specialty without understanding the general significance and meaning of that which gave it birth and continues to give sustenance?

Generalizations, one is told, are dangerous. So is life, for that matter, and it is built upon generalizations—from the earliest effort of the adventurer who dared to eat a second berry because the first had not killed him. So I will stick to my generalizing. . . .*

Most of the students who major in physical education intend to teach and/or coach and they are often confused by the interrelationships among the fields of physical education, health education, and recreation. Added to this confusion is the vexing problem of placing athletics in its proper perspective. Such perplexity may be nurtured by the limitations of the student's own experience and by the interpretation of these fields by the lay public. A perusal of the materials in this book should aid in ameliorating the dilemma.

All chapters contain updated references, most chapters are significantly revised, and two new chapters have been added: Philosophical Foundations, and Adult Fitness. In addition, the revised edition is divided into three main parts. Part I, The Discipline and Its Foundations, includes chapters on the foundational areas pertinent to physical education including philosophy, history, biomechanics, motor behavior, and physiology. Part II, Pedagogical Bases, includes those chapters which deal specifically with the profession of teaching and coaching. Part III, Physical Education and Allied Fields of Study, includes those chapters which attempt to show interrelationships among the allied fields.

ACKNOWLEDGMENTS

The authors wish to express appreciation to the following colleagues for reviewing the manuscript in their respective areas of specialty: Ronald Bos, Heidie Mitchell, Larry Golding, Grace Figley, Shirley Van Valkenburg, Robert Stadulis, Betty Hartman, and Dorothy Zakrajsek.

Kent, Ohio   B. L. S.
November 1977   M. C. R.

---

* Freya Stark, *The Lycian Shore* (New York: Harcourt, Brace & World, 1956), p. 103.

Contents

Part I
The Discipline
and
Its Foundations

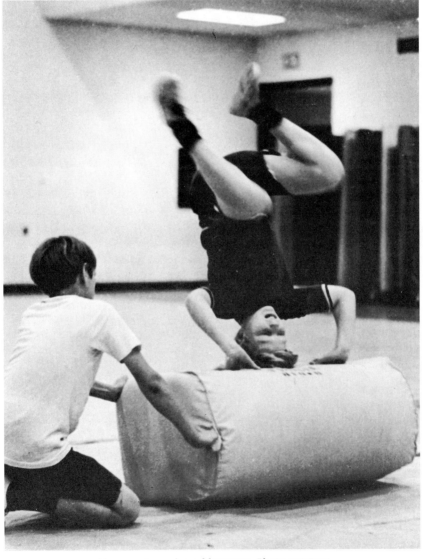

Movement, a universal language. Photo courtesy
of Lorie Coll and Ravenna (Ohio) City School System.

Chapter 1
Physical Education, a Discipline

Almost all really new ideas have a certain aspect of foolishness when they are first produced, and almost any idea which jogs you out of your current abstractions may be better than nothing.

ALFRED NORTH WHITEHEAD

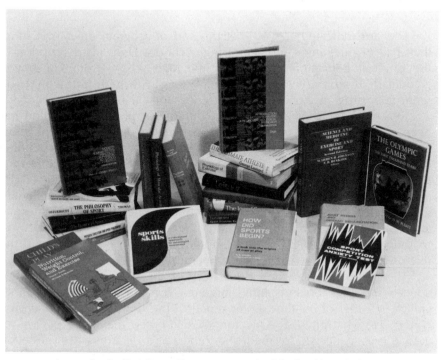

An academic discipline relies on an organized body of knowledge.

GEORGE LEONARD, author of *The Ultimate Athlete* and a critic of traditional physical education and competitive athletic programs in the schools of the United States, characterized the typical "gym class" as follows:

> The class period begins with students scrambling to change into gym clothes, then standing for a quasi-military dress inspection. The military sensibility continues to hold sway through five or ten minutes of calisthenics—push-ups, sit-ups, jumping jacks, toe touches, knee bends. Students may then be ordered to run a lap around the track, though running laps is in some cases reserved by the instructor for use as a punishment. After this, discipline goes rather rapidly downhill as students move on to the game of the day—softball, volleyball, flag football, field hockey, basketball. Play is sometimes preceded by a brief status-confirmation ritual known as "choosing sides." What with all of this, there is little time for the game itself. Students have yet one more ritual ahead of them: the shower. So much attention is devoted to this activity, in fact, that it might be seen by an anthropologist as the *raison d'être* of traditional physical education; in some schools students are inspected as they leave the shower room, ostensibly to make sure they are wet all over. Needless to say, boys' classes are separate from girls'.[1]

Leonard indicated as well that this sort of program prevails in more than half of our junior and senior high schools. Does his description fit the physical education program in the high school from which you graduated? If so, do you see anything wrong with it? If not, would you judge your program to have been better or worse than the one described?

Regardless of your answers, be assured that physical education has been an enigma for many years and to many people. At present, most people variously conceive of physical education as a muscle-building cult, as interscholastic athletics, or as a play period. To some educators, physical education is a nonintellectual class, unworthy of academic credit, in "gym." The freshman physical education major, cherishing pleasant memories of classes and sports competition conducted in an informal atmosphere under vibrant and youthful leadership, often looks forward to four years of preparation in "fun and games" in order to spend the rest of his or her life reliving those memories.

The confusion regarding the nature of the work done by physical education professionals is long-standing. Nearly a century ago, Luther Gulick, a leader of his time, complained of the general misapprehension concerning what physical educators do. He noted that some people regarded it as a specialty of medicine, others as a department of athletics, and still others as the process of building up muscular tissue.[2] Even today professional physical educators do not uniformly agree on a definition of physical education, much less on the objectives of the field or on its place in the total educational spectrum. Little wonder, then, that the perplexity exists.

But times are changing! There is strong evidence that the American Academy of Physical Education, among other groups and individuals, has given birth to a commitment toward formulating a theoretical framework of physical education that is not only empirically valid but also functional —a theoretical framework that, once formulated, not only will be acceptable to all those who labor as physical educators but will also, let us hope, guide them toward program excellence. The beginnings were painful, primarily because no one had ever before truly wrestled with the problem of delineating a body of knowledge in physical education, but the product is healthy and it is growing mightily, nurtured by dedicated scholar-teacher researchers as they scientifically explore the phenomena of people, movement, and meaning. In fact, the chairperson of the Scholarly Directions Committee, in an address to the Alliance for Health, Physical Education, and Recreation membership at large, indicated that the primary concern of the committee is to encourage scholars to extend the "horizons, boundaries, and dimensions" of basic knowledge in physical education and to organize that knowledge in such a way as to serve to generate new knowledge.[3]

The purpose of this chapter, then, is to discuss physical education as a discipline in order that the prospective physical educator can gain some insight into the intricate, diverse, and yet unified body of knowledge currently entitled physical education.

WHAT'S IN A NAME?

Terminology and semantics have played significant roles in creating and promoting the confusion noted in our field. The school program in what we now call *physical education* was probably first called *physical culture* in this country. That term undoubtedly referred to an emphasis on the development of the "body beautiful" through gymnastic exercises, conducted to music, which stressed rhythm and grace. Its use was questioned with the advent, in the early twentieth century, of the "new" system of physical education—a system which stressed the natural activities of games and dance rather than the more formal gymnastic exercises. Today, although the term "physical culture" is still used on occasion by the nonprofessional when discussing the field of physical education, it is largely identified with body-building cults.

Physical training was the term adopted when there was a shift to organic fitness, as espoused by such early leaders in the field as Edward Hitchcock and Dudley Allen Sargent. Although that term also fell into disrepute, it has never ceased to be used by some agencies, notably the military. When used in this context, it continues to imply an almost exclusive emphasis on physical fitness for a specific purpose, such as military preparedness or a particular athletic event.

Early in the twentieth century there was a shift to educational objectives when such leaders as Luther Gulick, Thomas Wood, and Clark Hetherington popularized the phrase "education *through* the physical." In fact, it is interesting to note that the objectives for physical education as proposed by Hetherington at that time not only are acceptable today, but are, in fact, the objectives embraced by many current physical educators. Since these leaders were dedicated to making the field more educational, its name quite naturally emerged as *physical education*.

Uncertainty in meaning still characterizes many of the terms we use. Just what does *physical fitness* connote? What are the differences between *movement education* and *basic movement*? Are *motor learning* and *motor behavior* synonymous terms? Are there real distinctions among *play, games, sports,* and *athletics*?

Adding to the confusion is the fact that, in this jet age, travel between continents and international exchange programs are commonplace. Thus the difference in terms and their meaning in other areas of the world becomes a factor. Some foreign countries continue to call their programs physical culture or physical training. What is *football* in Great Britain is *soccer* in the United States; likewise, their *educational gymnastics* is our *movement education*. *Gymnastics* in some European countries is what we call *physical education* in this country, and their *athletics* is equivalent to our *track and field*.

Current scholars in physical education are questioning the appropriateness of the title of the field as they consider whether or not physical education is a discipline with an organized body of knowledge and as they espouse a need to consider the theoretical rather than to concentrate almost exclusively on the practical. To many of these scholars, the term is not only limiting but offensive as well. Still, some of the proposed designations, such as ergonomics, kinesiology, biokinetics, movement education, anthropokinesiology, and exercise physiology, seem also to be unacceptable because upon analysis, they seem ambiguous or limited. Regardless of the rubric, there seems to be general consensus that the field is primarily concerned with human movement and all its ramifications—physical, psychological, sociological, and philosophic.

Just as the title of the field has changed from time to time, so has its definition. Such definitions have run the gamut from the nebulous "physical education is education through the physical" to quite precise delineations of objectives, programs, and other aspects. One of the most recent definitions, which seems to be gaining acceptance throughout the country and is the one advanced by the authors of this book, is *physical education is the art and science of human movement*. (This definition should not in any way be considered synonymous with the "movement movement." Movement education is but one part of the total physical education program, and its role is discussed in detail in Chapter 8.) In order to illuminate this definition, we will now examine it briefly.

When the *art* of movement is considered, the aesthetic quality of any skilled, graceful movement is involved—whether it is the dancer executing leaps and turns, the football player blocking an opponent, or the youngster skipping rope. The *science* of movement is employed by the track coach when he or she explains to a discus thrower the role of the body's center of gravity in relation to force and body levels, by the research professor as he or she measures maximum oxygen uptake during strenuous exercise, or by the swimming teacher as he or she applies Newton's third law of motion to an analysis of the flutter kick.

WHAT IS A DISCIPLINE?

Is Physical Education a Discipline?

Many scholars have been concerned with defining and characterizing an academic discipline. Just as such scholars as Philip Phenix, Joseph Schwab, Benjamin Bloom, and Jerome Bruner have wrestled with the task of generally delineating the necessary components of a discipline and its basic body of knowledge, so, too, have such physical educators as Franklin Henry, John Nixon, Warren Fraleigh, G. Lawrence Rarick, Ruth Abernathy, Gerald Kenyon, Aileene Lockhart, and Earle Zeigler been concerned with a specific formulation of the discipline of physical education.

Beginning in 1964 with articles by Abernathy and Waltz,[4] Lockhart,[5] and Henry,[6] through an entire issue of *Quest*[7] devoted to the subject in 1967, to a most cogent treatise by Kenyon[8] in 1968, and a "disciplinary" definition of sport by Zeigler[9] in 1976, many thoughtful as well as thought-provoking commentaries have been written on the subject. There is, of course, no universal consensus on whether physical education is or is not a discipline and, if it is, what its peculiar foci are. No doubt these issues will continue to be debated by perceptive scholars of physical education, both students and faculty. In an attempt to answer this question, physical educators must be concerned with a definition of a discipline, together with applicable criteria.

In the meantime, no one can deny that we have a considerable body of knowledge that is important to our field. That knowledge consists of facts and principles from many cognate fields, such as physiology, anthropology, philosophy, psychology, sociology, biology, history, and physics. This fact does not negate the idea that *physical education* has a body of knowledge, since a body of knowledge can be—and indeed usually is—interdisciplinary in nature. In physical education, however, much of the knowledge underlying the discipline has been unstructured, and, just as there has been, perhaps, too little concern with the generation of new knowledge, there definitely has been too little concern with transmitting such knowledge to prospective teachers, as well as to teachers in the field. We have been too preoccupied with teaching prospective teachers *what* they will teach on entering the field and *how* it should be taught. Actually, a discipline is little concerned with how the knowledge is used; nevertheless, if we organize our considerable knowledge and transmit it to prospective teachers more effectively, they in turn should be better prepared to teach the *why* of physical education and thus become educators in stead of merely skilled practitioners.

According to Henry:

> An academic discipline is an organized body of knowledge collectively embraced in a formal course of learning. The acquisition of such knowledge is assumed to be an adequate and worthy objective as such, without any demonstration or requirement of practical application. The content is theoretical and scholarly as distinguished from technical and professional.[10]

A definition as such does not tell us whether physical education is a discipline. We can say, for example, that we have "theoretical, scholarly content" but do we use such knowledge? Accordingly, it is well to apply some criteria to ascertain how well we meet them. Nixon, after reviewing several authorities who wrote generally on the subject of identifying and describing the criteria that must be met before a field of study can rightfully call itself a discipline, summarized and categorized the various criteria around "seven distinguishable elements," as follows:

1. A discipline has an identifiable domain; it asks vital questions; it deals with immensely significant themes, a specifiable scope of inquiry, a central core of interest; it has a definite beginning point; and it has stated goals.

2. A discipline is characterized by a substantial history and a publicly recognized tradition exemplified by time-tested works.

3. A discipline is rooted in an appropriate structure; it has its unique conceptual structure, and it employs a syntactical structure; the structure organizes a body of imposed conceptions (basic concepts); and it consists of conceptual relationships as well as appropriate relations between fact.

4. A discipline possesses a unique integrity and arbitrary quality.

5. A discipline is recognized by the procedures and methods it employs; it utilizes intellectual and conceptual tools as well as technical and mechanical tools; it follows a relevant set of rules; it is recognized by its basic set of procedures, all of which lead to ways of learning and knowing in the domain of the discipline.

6. A discipline is recognized as a process as well as noted for its products (knowledge, principles, generalizations).

7. Finally, a discipline relies on accurate language, a participants' language, to provide precise, careful communication both within its ranks and to outsiders.[11]

The mere listing of such criteria does not answer the question of whether or not physical education can rightfully be called a discipline. The criteria must somehow be applied. Thoughtful faculty members can wrestle with such application; but so, too, can thoughtful professional students in physical education—graduate or undergraduate, doctoral candidate or freshman.

DISCIPLINE OR PROFESSION?

A later chapter in this book concerns itself with the "profession" of physical education and with the "professional" people within the field. It is therefore appropriate at this point to state only that a discipline is not synonymous with a profession. Kenyon emphasizes that one of the objectives of a discipline is to understand some portion of reality, whereas one of the prime goals of a profession is to make needed alterations in reality in order to improve humanity.

> If a discipline has curiosity as its motivation, a profession has as its motive service, i.e., the welfare of humanity. It is simply a matter of "what is" vs. "what ought to be." It follows, therefore, that arguing that a given field can be simultaneously a profession and a discipline is little else save a logically invalid contradiction of terms. The only solution to this dilemma, as I see it, is to recognize that, while it is possible for the same phenomenon to serve as the focal point of both a profession and a discipline (subject matter for one, a medium for the other), it is there that the similarity ends. Thus, the expression "physical education" with its obvious professional connotations, is not a suitable label for both the profession and disciplinary aspects of human physical activity. However, because of its widespread currency, and despite the semantic difficulties long alluded to, the term might be retained, but in a restricted sense. Those who would use physical activity to change behavior—whether it be cognitive, affective or psychomotor—I would call physical educators. On the other hand, those whose objective it is to understand the phenomenon, I would consider members of a discipline, the name of which is still the topic of much debate.[12]

It is thus apparent, at least in the minds of many current leaders, that physical education as an academic discipline is based on an organized body of knowledge concerning human movement and that one must understand this body of knowledge before one can learn to transmit understanding to others via the profession of teaching. Fraleigh discusses this tenet succinctly.

> ... it is now appropriate to say that understanding the nature of the subject matter precedes in time the attempt to study educational

process either in or through the subject matter. Thus, in teacher education conscious study to understand the phenomena of vigorous human movement precedes in time conscious study to understand the process of education in and/or through vigorous human movement. The following premises tend to support this contention.

1. Depth of understanding of subject matter is a necessary prerequisite to intelligent attempts to transmit it to others.
2. Understanding the phenomenon of vigorous human movement is not exactly the same as understanding the process of teaching in and/or through vigorous human movement.
3. The perspective with which a learner and a teacher approach the study of subject matter has a great deal to do with what kind of understandings come out of that study.
4. Disciplined subject matter suggests by its nature appropriate methods of inquiry to investigate it. Methods of inquiry of a discipline must be carefully integrated with educational process in the form of instructional theory in order for effective learning to occur. Therefore, the presence of a disciplined subject matter is a prior necessity to study of integration of educational process with the subject matter.

Granted the validity of these assertions, the importance of formulating the subject matter of physical education into an academic discipline becomes apparent.[13]

The focus of this book is on the premise that there is a body of knowledge concerning human movement and that students who are just commencing their professional study in physical education need to be exposed to such knowledge as quickly as possible. Accordingly, an attempt is made to cite the latest research and to acquaint students with the vast number of library resources available in the field. We hope that, by the end of the course, students will be better prepared to make at least a tentative decision on which of the many avenues available to them in physical education they may wish to choose. Teacher? Researcher? Coach? Dancer? Curriculum expert? Administrator? Athletic trainer? Sports performer? YMCA or YWCA director? Spa owner? Physical therapist?

Regardless of the answers reached to the questions raised in this chapter, one cannot escape the truism that "actions speak louder than words." If physical education is an academic discipline, the implications for the field seem clear. As discussed above, we must do a better, more thorough job of teaching the body of knowledge basic to the discipline to those students who are pursuing physical education as a college major regardless of their intended vocational use of such knowledge. Since presently a large majority of those studying physical education wish to teach and coach and since it is at the grass-roots level of public educa-

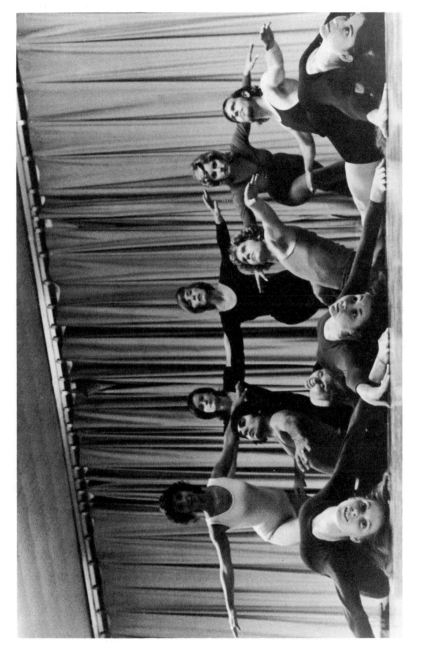

Dance, one form of human movement. Photo courtesy of Department of Physical Education, Kent State University.

tion where the discipline must be more carefully delineated to all students if the profession of physical education is to be advanced, competent teachers—teachers who not only understand the *whys* of their profession but also know how to construct sound school programs in physical education and how to organize efficiently so that the *hows* and *whats* are more adequately effectuated.

In the long run, the entire future of physical education rests on the shoulders of those whose vocation it is. They must be respected by their administrators, their colleagues, their students, and their public. Quality in every aspect of the discipline is the only answer to the ultimate attainment of prestige.

STUDENT PROJECTS

1. Obtain biographical information on the leaders in the field, past and present, who were named in this chapter. What names might be added to the list?
2. Apply Nixon's criteria regarding a discipline to physical education, decide how well physical education meets each one, and justify your decision.
3. What objectives for physical education did Clark Hetherington propose? Why are they still applicable today?
4. Are other countries in the world concerned about physical education becoming an academic discipline? Make a list of selected countries which are concerned and those which are not. Try to theorize why.
5. What basic library research tools are housed in your university library? Why might it be desirable to make a list of them, together with their call numbers and the specific purpose each serves?
6. Prepare oral and/or written reports on specific resources from the periodicals in the references at the end of the chapter.
7. Survey some of the nonphysical education majors in your residence hall to ascertain how they define physical education. Ask them to describe their high school physical education program.
8. Is an organized program of athletics an integral part of physical education? Defend your answer.

GLOSSARY OF TERMS

Physical culture A theory of physical activity which has as its basis the promotion of body development.

Physical training Use of physical exercise for preparation to participate in a specific activity or sport.

Physical education   The art and science of human movement.

Intramurals   Recreation activities carried on within an institution (school).

Extramurals   The extension of the intramural program to include other schools.

Discipline   An area of study characterized by an organized body of knowledge.

Profession   The practice of a discipline within a defined context, such as a code of ethics.

"Gym"   A commonly heard label for the school program in physical education, the use of which should be discouraged. It denotes only the place in which the program is conducted and does not properly refer to the program itself.

REFERENCES

1. George Leonard, "Why Johnny Can't Run," *The Atlantic*, August 1975, 55–56. Reprinted by permission of The Viking Press, Inc., © 1974.

2. Luther Gulick, "Physical Education: A New Profession," *Proceedings*, American Association for the Advancement of Physical Education, 1890, p. 59.

3. W. R. Morford, "New Frontiers in Physical Education: The Need for Scholarship" (Paper presented at the national conference of the AAHPER, Seattle, Washington, April 1970).

4. Ruth Abernathy and Maryann Waltz, "Toward a Discipline: First Steps First," *Quest* **2** (April 1964), pp. 1–7.

5. Aileene Lockhart, "What's in a Name?" *Quest* **2** (April 1964), pp. 9–13.

6. Franklin M. Henry, "Physical Education: An Academic Discipline," *JOHPER* 37 (September 1964), pp. 32–33, 69.

7. *Quest* **9** (December 1967).

8. Gerald S. Kenyon, "On the Conceptualization of Sub-Disciplines Within an Academic Discipline Dealing with Human Movement," *Proceedings*, National College Physical Education Association for Men (1968), pp. 34–45.

9. Earle F. Zeigler, "A Model for the Optimum Development of a Social Force Known as Sport." *International Journal of Physical Education* **XIII** (Spring 1976), pp. 11–17.

10. Henry, p. 32.

11. John E. Nixon, "The Criteria of a Discipline," *Quest* **9** (December 1967), p. 47.

12. Gerald S. Kenyon, "A Sociology of Sport: On Becoming a Sub-Discipline," in *New Perspectives of Man in Action*, eds. R. C. Brown and B. J. Cratty (Englewood Cliffs, N.J.: Prentice-Hall, 1969), p. 165.

13. Warren P. Fraleigh, "Toward a Conceptual Model of the Academic Subject Matter of Physical Education as a Discipline," *Proceedings*, National College Physical Education Association for Men (1967), p. 32.

SELECTED READINGS

Abernathy, Ruth, and Waltz, Maryann. "Toward a Discipline: First Steps First." *Quest* **2** (April 1964), pp. 1–7.

Bloom, Benjamin S., ed. *Taxonomy of Educational Objectives*. New York: Longmans, Green, 1956.

Brackenbury, Robert L. "Physical Education, an Intellectual Emphasis?" *Quest* **1** (December 1963), pp. 3–6.

Bruner, Jerome S. *Toward a Theory of Instruction*. Cambridge: Harvard University Press, 1966.

Elam, S., ed. *Education and the Structure of Knowledge*. Chicago: Rand McNally, 1964.

Felshin, Jan. *More Than Movement*. Philadelphia: Lea & Febiger, 1972.

Flaten, Clarence. Physical Education as Inquiry," *Conference Proceedings*, Midwest Association of Physical Education for College Women (October 1969), pp. 35–36.

Fraleigh, Warren P. "Toward a Conceptual Model of the Academic Subject Matter of Physical Education as a Discipline." *Proceedings*, National College Physical Education Association for Men (1966), pp. 31–39.

———. A Prologue to the Study of Theory Building in Physical Education." *Quest* **12** (May 1969), pp. 26–33.

Gulick, Luther. "Physical Education: A New Profession." *Proceedings*, American Association for the Advancement of Physical Education (1890), p. 59

Henry, Franklin M. "Physical Education: An Academic Discipline." *Journal of Health, Physical Education and Recreation* **37** (September 1964), pp. 32–33, 69.

Hill, J. M., ed. *The Body of Knowledge Unique to the Profession of Education*. Washington: Pi Lambda Theta, 1966.

Jewett, Ann. "Implications from Curriculum Theory for Physical Education." *American Academy of Physical Education Papers* **2** (October 1968).

Kenyon, Gerald S. "On the Conceptualization of Sub-Disciplines Within an Academic Discipline Dealing with Human Movement." *Proceedings*, National College Physical Education Association for Men (1968), pp. 34–45.

———. "A Sociology of Sport: On Becoming a Sub-Discipline." In *New Perspectives of Man in Action*, edited by R. C. Brown and B. J. Cratty. pp. 163–180. Englewood Cliffs, N.J.: Prentice-Hall, 1969.

Kroll, Walter. *Perspectives in Physical Education*. New York: Academic Press, 1971.

Larson, Leonard A. "Professional Preparation for the Activity Sciences. *Journal of Sports Medicine* **5** (March 1965), pp. 15–22.

Leonard, George. *The Ultimate Athlete*. New York: Viking, 1974.

———. "Why Johnny Can't Run." *The Atlantic*, 236:2 (August 1975), 55–60.

Lockhart, Aileene. "What's in a Name?" *Quest* **2** (April 1964), pp. 9–13.

MacKenzie, Marlin M. *Toward a New Curriculum in Physical Education*. New York: McGraw-Hill, 1969.

Metheny, Eleanor. "The 'Design' Conference." *Journal of Health, Physical Education and Recreation* **37** (May 1966), p. 6.

Mosston, Muska. *Teaching Physical Education.* Columbus, Ohio: Charles E. Merrill, 1966.

Mosston, Muska, and Mueller, Rudy. "Mission, Omission and Submission in Physical Education." *Proceedings,* NCPEAM, 1970, pp. 122–130.

Olsen, A. Morgan. "On the Elaboration of Physical Education Theory." *Proceedings,* International Seminar on Research in Physical Education in Universities and Colleges, Paris, 1966.

Paddick, Robert J. "The Nature and Place of a Field of Knowledge in Physical Education." Master's thesis, University of Alberta, 1967.

Quest **9** (December 1967). Entire issue.

Report of the National Conference on Interpretation of Physical Education. Chicago: Athletic Institute, 1961.

Siedentop, Daryl. *Physical Education: Introductory Analysis.* Dubuque, Iowa: W. C. Brown, 1976.

Smith, Karl U. "Cybernetic Foundations of Physical Behavioral Science." *Quest* **7** (May 1967), pp. 26–82.

Turner, Edward T. "Physical Education: A Paradoxical Phenomenon." *The Physical Educator* **25** (December 1968), pp. 174–176.

Singer, Robert, ed. *Physical Education: Foundations.* New York: Holt, Rinehart and Winston, 1976.

Ulrich, Celeste, and Nixon, John, eds. *Tones of Theory.* Washington, D.C.: AAHPER, 1972.

Zeigler, Earle E. "A Model for the Optimum Development of a Social Force Known as Sport." *International Journal of Physical Education* **XIII** (Spring 1976).

Chapter 2
Our Legacy from the Past

Those who cannot remember the past are condemned to repeat it.

SANTAYANA

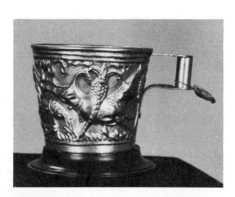

**Mycenean cup
(1300–1100 B.C.)**

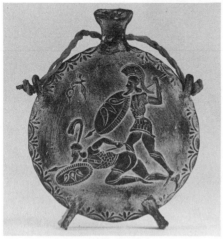

Amphora (container for oil for athletes)

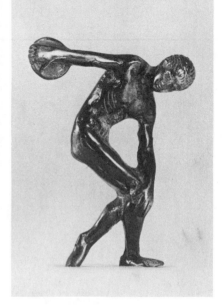

Diskobolus **by Myron** ▶

INTRODUCTION

FROM past to present, physical education has been an index of society—neither better nor worse than other aspects of society. Physical education has been used to bring people together for noble purposes, to indicate the virility of a nation, and unfortunately, to get citizens ready to defend themselves and their countries and, in the last analysis, to destroy each other. Since physical education is adaptable, it has been used and misused by the leaders of the past. The recent invitation to the United States Table Tennis Team to visit Red China in April 1971 was hailed around the world as a fine diplomatic move and the first step in the renewal of direct relations between Red China and the United States. As expressed by one commentator, the "Great Wall of China now has a hole in it the size of a ping pong ball."

The philosophies, ethics, customs, and even the economic conditions of the people of the times have been reflected through the medium of physical education and sports. As an example of the reflection of economic conditions, some of the more popular sports during the Depression of the 1930s, such as volleyball, fishing, and softball (without gloves), were those in which the equipment, though expendable, was long-lasting. In periods of affluence, boating, golf, bowling, and drag racing are among the more popular activities.

A study of the history of physical education and sports also shows that a decline in sports participation is often an accompaniment of moral decay and a harbinger of the decline of a culture. For example, sports scandals are not a product of this age alone. "Spectatoritis"—the increased dependence of peoples on others' participating for them—became in itself a sign of what lay ahead. This was true in Egypt, in later Greek periods, in Rome—and it is true today.

In any culture, the type of physical education and sports is influenced by the climate and the geographic location, by the physical characteristics of the people, and by the dominant religion. Throughout history, religion has both encouraged and impeded the physical activity of people. A number of our physical education activities and sports had their origins in religious ceremonies.

Although it is impossible to treat more than sketchily the history of physical education in one unit of an introductory textbook, the authors wish to give students some insights into their heritage. The programs in this country are eclectic in nature, and their roots lie in many foreign countries. Consequently, some of the problems we have are the result of adapting foreign systems of physical education to our own programs. It is the authors' hope that at a later stage of professional preparation students will study the history of physical education in greater detail in order better to understand present programs.

PRIMITIVE HUMAN CULTURES

Although preceded by Solo, Rhodesian, and Neanderthal peoples, the Cro-Magnon remains are the source of most of the information we have of primitive peoples. They replaced the Neanderthals in Europe and seem to have colonized the world. They left the world their cave paintings, stone engravings, and carved figures. Much of their education was physical since they were both hunters and hunted. Their education was geared strictly to survival as they learned to obtain food and water and to repel their enemies. Their civilization was not inherited genetically. They had to learn it and pass it on to those that followed. At first they traveled to find new sources of food. They lived by hunting, fishing, and gathering plants. Later they domesticated animals to make their travel easier. As they learned to grow food, they traveled less and developed their family, clan, and society. The clay of the earth, hardened by fire, became the first all-weather playground for their children.

Except for those events necessary for survival, dance was probably the activity in which most adult men participated. When and how early peoples began to dance is a matter of conjecture. We know that in most cultures dance was performed mostly by the males, as it is in the primitive tribes still on earth today. Among the "dawn people" of the Kalapalo Indians, who live along the Amazon in Central Brazil, this tradition is still carried on, untouched by civilization. They danced to placate the gods, to bring rain, to cure the sick, and to bury the dead. They danced in "sympathetic magic"; that is, by pantomime to suggest a result they hoped would occur. If they needed meat, they pantomimed the hunt and the kill. If they needed rain, they pantomimed the flowing clouds and falling rain drops. Primitive peoples could not distinguish between magic and science. They laid the groundwork for what would be recorded as history later. Their survival activities became recreational in nature for future cultures.

THE FAR EAST

Although some think of the Far East as being the seat of the most ancient civilizations, the recorded history of the area does not support this assumption. Future archaeological findings may reveal the facts. The Far East had practically no impact on our physical education programs in the past, but at the present some Eastern combative activities are being added to the curriculum. Empty-hand combat was the principal contribution of the ancient Far East to the present.

India

There has been a paucity of physical education and sports activities among the people of India. The military motive was nonexistent since the oceans and the mountains protected the people from other warlike nations, except for a few short-lived intrusions (that of Alexander the Great, for example). The hot, humid climate was not conducive to vigorous activity. Furthermore, the basic religion, Hinduism, did not encourage such activities. Finally, problems of famine and sanitation prevented any large-scale participation since the ill and the starving were disinclined to participate.

The art of yoga may have been the one outstanding Indian contribution to physical activity—although it may be difficult to fit that practice into any definition of "activity." Former claims that badminton originated in India are no longer accepted since there is ample evidence that it was brought to India by the British colonists. India has experienced some degree of success internationally in soccer and field hockey.

China

The climate of China, unlike that of India, was conducive to participation in physical activity. Although the entire area had natural boundaries, such as the mountains and the sea, the feudal wars of the pre-Christian period gave the ruling classes the motive for learning combative sports. The Great Wall, built during the Chin Dynasty, was intended to protect China from its land-based enemies to the west and north.

As early as 2600 B.C., there were evidences of a system of "medical gymnastics," the first adapted and corrective physical education programs in history. Kite-flying also had its origin in China and was an activity of both children and adults. It took the form of a combative sport when devices were added to cut the strings of other kite flyers. Head-butting satisfied the most bloodthirsty fan; two participants donned the skulls or horns of animals and then ran headlong into each other until one was unconscious.

The early Chinese also had boxing in many forms, but their greatest single contribution was the development of jiu-jitsu. Jiu-jitsu and other empty-handed methods of combat were practiced by Chinese monks to thwart bandits since the monks were forbidden to carry arms. Empty-handed methods of combat were exported to Japan, Korea, and other parts of the Far East, where they were refined to fit the needs and desires of the people. Judo and karate are examples of this development. Although forms of soccer were played in many cultures, the Chinese played a one-goal game of soccer with a ball made of eight conical pieces of leather. Goals were a series of holes dug in the ends of the playing areas.

Japan

Although the modern Japanese are among the most enthusiastic sports participants and spectators in the world, their contribution to physical education and sports in the past were meager. Much of their culture was influenced by the Chinese, and so were their physical activities. They perfected the arts of judo and karate and spread these activities to other countries. Since their civilization was characterized by the feudal system for a long period of time, only the ruling or warrior classes participated in physical education and sports. Among the martial arts were fencing, archery on horseback, and wrestling. The nobility also hunted with hawks.

THE MIDDLE EAST

The cradle of civilization, whose peoples included the Eygptians, Assyrians, Babylonians, Sumarians, and Hebrews, was also the cradle of physical education. In all of these cultures, the military motive was present and the spirit of the people was conductive to an active life. Much of the male adult's time was spent in military service, labor, or sports. In the early history of these cultures, women were relegated to a minor role. A notable exception was the early Egyptian woman, who enjoyed full freedom and status comparable to that of the Egyptian man.

Among the physical activities of the Egyptians were horsemanship, hunting, and swimming. The last was considered vital in that a swimming accident might dictate a watery grave rather than the tomb burial that was so important in their religion. In Egypt the nobleman rarely danced except for religious ceremonies. Dancing was performed either by his slaves or by professional dancers. Other sports were wrestling, bullfighting, acrobatics, and some ball games, including a version of keep-away with a ball. The person dropping the ball became the "donkey."

The Hebrew contribution was principally in the realm of health; the practice of handwashing and the dietary laws had both religious and health connotations. The activities mentioned previously also applied to the Jewish people. Swimming as an activity was referred to in the Bible by the prophet Isaiah: "And he shall stretch forth his hands under him, as he that swimmeth stretcheth forth his hands to swim . . ." (Isa. 23:11).

Persia

Persia deserves special consideration for several reasons, not the least of which is the fact that Persian culture served as the connection between Western culture and the Far East. The Persians were also the first people to offer an organized program of physical activities for a segment of their population. At age six, the boys were taken over by the state to be trained for the military. They were taught to shoot, to ride, and to speak the truth, and their activities included swimming, horseback riding, archery, throwing the javelin, and using the slingshot.

As in the other countries about them, the women were kept in seclusion. Persians did not dance themselves; their entertainment came from professional dancers.

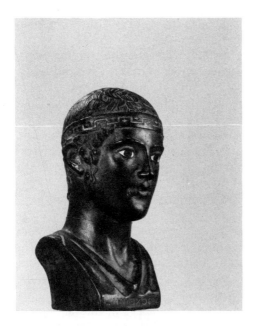

ΗΝΙΟΧΟΣ **The Charioteer of Delphi 478 B.C.**

One of the weaknesses of Persia as a culture was its lack of general education; the emphasis was on physical education only. This weakness constituted a reverse form of the practice of separating the training of the mind and body, a distinct dichotomy. Physical educationists today decry the dichotomy of mind and body and insist that education includes more than merely the mind. By the same token, the reversed emphasis on the body, as practiced in Persia, was not educationally sound.

GREEK PHYSICAL EDUCATION

No country before the time of ancient Greece ever held sports and physical activity in greater regard and no country since has matched the ancient Greeks in their enthusiasm. From the time of the Minoan period in Crete until the Roman conquest of Greece, physical activity held a prominent place. Cretan sports included boxing, wrestling, running, bull-fighting, and acrobatic bull-leaping. Women were both spectators and participants, especially in the art of bull-leaping, in which participants vaulted or tumbled over a charging bull. Artifacts suggest the superiority of boxing styles of the Minoan period over those of later Greek periods.

During the Homeric period, all warriors were supposed to be athletes. Some of their contests, included in the funeral games in honor of Patroclus, are described in the *Iliad*. The events were chariot race, boxing, and wrestling; such prizes as a woman's skilled handiwork, a mare in foal, and golden two-handled urns were awarded. These and other events are described in the *Odyssey*.

The city-state system promoted the development of the athletic festival, which later developed into the Olympic or Pan-Hellenic games. Physical education and athletics held different status in the different city-states. The divergence may be noted in an examination of Sparta and Athens. In warlike Sparta a small group of citizens controlled the slaves who worked the fields and produced goods. Boys of seven were taken by the state and trained to rule through military might. Swimming, wrestling, running, and jumping were the stressed activities. Girls between seven and seventeen followed a similar regimen, because the Spartans considered vigorous activity as preparation for living. There was very little cultural or general education for the citizen of Sparta. Male citizens stayed in the military until retirement at about the age of fifty.

Athens is an example of the ideal city-state. There was a balance between preparation for the military and preparation for the social, political, and religious life of the state. Children played at ball, swings, and hoops, as children do today. Young women remained in semiseclusion while preparing to take their places in the family structure. Young men were educated in both body and mind, studying such subjects as grammar, music, and gymnastics. The gymnasium (merely a playfield) and palaestra (wrestling areas) were in evidence everywhere. Even in the later periods, when sports were criticized by philosophers and writers, gymnastics (physical education) was still well received.

Pan-Hellenic Games

The forerunner of our present Olympics began before the ninth century B.C. The most commonly accepted date of the first Olympic games is 776 B.C. They were conducted for the citizens of the city-states as individuals; team scores were not kept. Games at four principal locations and many lesser ones were scheduled around those held at Olympia near the plain of Elis. The games held at Delphi, Corinth, and Nemea were the most widely known.

The eligibility rules for these contests, some of which are similar to rules for athletic conferences today, included the following.

1. Participants had to be of pure Greek stock.
2. Participants might never have committed a crime.
3. Females were not allowed to participate or to watch.
4. Participants must have practiced a specified period of time (about nine months).
5. Once they had entered, participants were not allowed to withdraw.
6. There were only two classes of participation—men's and boy's—and there were no weight classifications.

The officials of the contests were elected by the citizens of the local community and wielded considerable power. During the training period, they could eliminate participants they found to be unfit or not sufficiently skilled for the games. There were no preliminary meets, but this procedure kept the participants to a workable number. Then, too, the winner was not always the one who ran the fastest or jumped the farthest. The judges voted for the winner on both his finish and his form. Finally, game officials were empowered to have participants physically beaten for false starts and illegal holds.

There were many things wrong with Greek games and athletics, and from them we should learn lessons that are applicable today. The Greeks had their own version of scandals and fixes. Judges accepted bribes to vote for athletes who were defeated, and participants bribed one another to perform poorly in events in order to permit others to win. (Nero was once awarded an olive crown even though he fell off his chariot.)

A change came to the games when the prizes took on monetary value and came to include even state subsidies for life. Professionalism developed because of both the increased value of the prizes and the increased length of training even for many "minor" games. Sports became a full-time occupation for the entire calendar year. Near the end of the Pan-Hellenic period, slaves were being trained to participate and represent the different city-states. The ordinary citizen became a spectator.

The various events were not greatly different from those of today. Boxing, wrestling, and track and field events were refined to the forms in which they were later adopted in subsequent cultures. The one exception was the sport of pankration, a combination of boxing, wrestling, and no-holds-barred brawling, in which only gouging and biting were illegal. Because the loser had to admit defeat, Spartans seldom took part in this event. A Spartan preferred death to admission of defeat. All activities were individual events and there were no team games in the Pan-Hellenic games.

ROMAN INFLUENCES

When Rome conquered Greece, it was itself conquered by the culture of Greece, including sports. Olympic-type games were carried on in most Roman provinces. At the same time that these sports were introduced to Rome, animal and blood sports were also introduced. The latter influenced the nature of other games, and brutality increased. Whereas boxers had formerly worn leather thongs, they now wore metal spikes that protruded in such a way as to cut up the opponent for the entertainment of the spectators. Chariot races were often won, not by the swiftest, but by the one who avoided the pitfalls of trickery.

Spectators increased in proportion to the brutality of the events. The participants were largely slaves, and the citizens sat as spectators in the large arenas. In the year 394 A.D., however, Emperor Theodosius, a

Christian, abolished the Olympics, and shortly afterward the last gladiatorial contests were held.

The large stadium for spectator viewing was among the contributions of the Roman culture to present-day sports. Gladiators were trained, housed, and fed in camps similar to our professional preseason football camps. One of the training camps for Roman gladiators was located in the city of Pompeii.

Women were allowed to attend although there was a period of time (during the reign of Augustus) when they could not attend until the late morning hours. At a still later period women participated as gladiators.

THE DARK AGES AND THE RENAISSANCE

After the fall of Rome, sports and physical education were of little or no importance. The Christian church emphasized the importance of the soul and the unimportance of the mortal body. Asceticism was diametrically opposed to physical activity other than work. During the Dark Ages, Christ and his disciples, who actually led robust lives, were portrayed with emaciated bodies and haggard faces.

Only the nobles received a good physical education. A nobleman's son had a choice of going into the clergy or becoming a knight. If he chose the latter, he started his training as a page (ages 7–14) and during that time learned the amenities of the court (eating, serving, using proper manners, and playing a musical instrument). Becoming a squire at age 14, he helped a knight with his equipment and duties while at the same time learning to ride, swim, use the sword, scale walls, and wage war. At the age of 21, the knight accepted his responsibility for protecting the land and the people of the realm from enemies. His was a full physical education, which included long training periods for tournaments and jousts. Much of our tournament conduct has been inherited from this period.

The Renaissance brought forth not only a rebirth of learning but also a renewed interest in the physical activities which contributed to a healthy body. Vergerius, Montaigne, Rabelais, Milton, Locke, and a host of others expressed themselves in writing concerning the need for physical education as well as for the training of the intellect. Most of them advocated a return to the Greek ideal of a balance between these two human aspects.

During the Reformation, some of the religious sects renounced any form of play or physical activity of a recreational nature. This development had an effect on physical education and sports in early America. The Puritans in America, by means of public censure of recreative activity and passage of "blue laws," did much to hamper the growth of physical education. One modern researcher, however, disagrees with many physical education historians on this point. Ballou challenges as implausible and unfounded the claim that the influence of asceticism was the major factor in the suppression of physical education. He suggests that Christianity condemned not physical activity per se but rather the improper use of it.[1]

GERMAN INFLUENCES

The most influential development in the German system of physical education was the *Turnverein* movement initiated by Frederick Jahn. Politically motivated, Jahn wanted to unite the small city-states of Germany into a powerful nation. A conventional teacher in the elementary schools, he taught physical education outside the schools in the late afternoons or on weekends. Later he met with the same boys in the summer periods and developed a system of leaders to assist him. Apparatus was constructed from tree trunks and other materials. The movement was questioned by government authorities since the unification it strove to accomplish threatened the rulers of the small city-states, and Jahn was arrested for his political activity. Released after two years, he was forbidden to live within ten miles of any city.

Adolph Spiess made many of Jahn's activities acceptable as part of the school program. In the meantime, many of Jahn's friends became political refugees in the United States and brought with them the *Turnverein* movement, which continued to affect programs in German ethnic neighborhoods of the Midwest even after its influence died in eastern colleges.

SWEDISH INFLUENCES

Per Henrick Ling, the founder of the Swedish system of physical education, was influenced by Franz Nachtegall of Denmark and Guts Muths of Germany. Ling's first interests were personal, because he sought benefits to an afflicted arm from fencing. His later program of strengthening exercises, free exercises, simple apparatus work, vaulting, and fencing was based on scientific principles of anatomy and physiology.

His successors, Branting and his own son, H. F. Ling, introduced gymnastics for girls and medical gymnastics. Equipment for these programs was devised to take care of large numbers of students at one time.

The Swedish system of physical education was introduced into the eastern United States, and at one time it constituted the official program in a number of eastern schools. Baron Nils Posse, who came to this country in 1885, was instrumental in having Mrs. Mary Hemenway, a Boston philanthropist, assemble the now famous Boston Conference of 1889 for the purpose of adopting Swedish gymnastics in the country's school systems. Historically, however, the greatest influence of the conference was the decision not to adopt any "system" of physical education. This conference is considered one of the milestones of American physical education.

BRITISH INFLUENCES

Except for a few periods in their history, the people of England have regularly favored sports and games over systems of formal physical education. Even when formal physical education classes were included in the school day, the after-school periods were devoted to games. Many of these games were developed in rural settings. The Englishman continued to play after his formal education was complete, and sports clubs arose to supply his need. This pattern is still characteristic of the English culture. The upper classes developed idealistic attitudes of amateurism, which stemmed from social behavior. The English concept of amateurism, promoted in most of England's colonial possessions, is the main source of inspiration for amateur codes in the United States. To this day, it has been difficult to resolve some of the current problems in the light of this definition of amateurism. The English definition of an amateur was socially based while our present one is financially based.

Many English games were brought to this country, and they form the nucleus of our present programs. Some, however, have been changed to such an extent that very little resemblance can now be noted. Examples are the evolution of football from soccer and rugby and baseball from cricket and rounders.

DOMESTIC INFLUENCES

Before the colonists came to the New World, the Indians, especially those of Central America, were developing civilizations as complex as those in Europe. In the ancient "Sun Kingdoms" of the Aztecs, Mayas, and Incas, there were dances and games that had been passed on for generations. One of those games had many of the elements of basketball. It was played all the way from Honduras to the region that is now our Southwest. The Aztecs called it *tlachtli,* and in the Mayan culture it was *pok-a-tok.* The ball was made of light, lively, but solid rubber. The goal was a vertical hoop made of stone and attached to a wall from ten to thirty feet above the ground. The players, who were not allowed to use their hands, tried to put the ball through the hoop with hips, head, or elbows. The spectator arrangement for this game, resembling the basketball arena of today, included courtside seats that were tiered for better viewing. Some historians feel that this sport is clearly an ancestor of the game later "invented" by Naismith.

When Europeans began to arrive in the New World, the very nature of the hostile environment dictated the colonial attitude toward sports and physical education activities. The people had to be fit to provide the food for their existence and to protect themselves from their enemies. Game and fish were plentiful, and the presence of both fresh and salt water promoted the activities of boating and swimming.

Although the religion dominant in most of the colonies frowned on sports, the settlers swam, fished, and hunted for pleasure as they found more leisure time. The men were each expected to give one day a month to the militia. The mornings were devoted to military affairs, but the afternoons were given over to races, wrestling, shooting, and other activities, including some "blood sports." One such blood sport involved having chained wild beasts fight each other or having a pack of dogs attack them. Another was the cockfight—an activity that has survived to this day although it is illegal in most states. Most blood sports did not survive, partly because hunting animals in their natural environment was inherently more interesting.

The introduction of slavery brought to this country a race of black people whose background of rhythm and dance influenced the dances of that time and has never ceased doing so. Our traders also watched Indians at play and learned their dances and some of their sports. The principal contribution of the Indians was the sport of lacrosse, first observed among the Canadian Indians.

As different systems of physical education were being introduced from Europe (Germany and Sweden), young people of this country were enjoying football, baseball, rowing, and other sports outside the jurisdiction of their schools. These sports had great meaning to the populace of a free and democratic society, and by the turn of the twentieth century, games and sports activities were supplanting formal systems of physical education in the schools.

CONCLUSIONS

Since the United States became a melting pot for emigrants from many parts of the world, physical education in this country is a blend of many forms of activity. With its roots in the past, it is nevertheless adaptable to changes in the nature of the culture. Wars, depressions, periods of inflation, and sedentary living have all contributed to the changing pattern of the programs. Conditions of the present will have an equally great impact on future programs.

It is imperative for the professional physical educator to identify those problems which have plagued the field since its inception in order that the mistakes of the past are not repeated. Some of our current problems have historical precedents. Among them are the trends toward (1) sedentary living by the affluent, (2) acting the role of spectator, either in person or via television, (3) removing the requirement of physical education from the schools, and (4) using sports and physical education as political or social weapons. These and other such problems have been dealt with in the past by other nations and cultures. Lessons already learned from these experiences need not be repeated again.

STUDENT PROJECTS

1. Select one of the cultures or time periods discussed in this chapter and report on its impact on present programs of physical education.
2. Examine the literature for information about the origins of ten modern sports, and report your findings. Include any discrepancies that you find interesting.

GLOSSARY OF TERMS

Medical gymnastics   Exercise for the prevention or correction of physical deviations.

Eclectic   Selecting what appears best from various systems.

"Blood sports"   Sports in which the participants (animals or men) fight until one has been physically beaten and is usually bleeding. Examples: bullfighting, cockfighting, bearbaiting, and boxing.

REFERENCES

1. Ralph B. Ballou, "An Analysis of the Writings of Selected Church Fathers to A.D. 394 to Reveal Attitudes Regarding Physical Activity" (Ph.D. diss., University of Oregon, 1965).

SELECTED READINGS

Ballou, Ralph. "An Analysis of the Writings of Selected Church Fathers to A.D. 394 to Reveal Attitudes Regarding Physical Activity." Ph.D. diss., University of Oregon, 1965.

Gardiner, E. Norman. *Athletics of the Ancient World*. Rev. ed. London: Oxford University Press, 1967.

Gerber, Ellen W. *Innovators and Institutions in Physical Education*. Philadelphia: Lea & Febiger, 1971.

Grupe, Ommo, ed. "Sport in Theological Perspective." In *The Scientific View of Sport*. Berlin: Springer-Verlag, 1972.

———. "Sport and Religions of the World." In *Sport in the Modern World*. Berlin: Springer-Verlag, 1973.

Harris, H. A. *Greek Athletes and Athletics*. London: Hutchison ,1964

Latourette, Kenneth Scott. *A Short History of the Far East*. 4th ed. New York: Macmillan, 1964.

Quest **11**, The National Association for Physical Education of College Women and the National College Physical Education Association for Men (December 1968).

Rice, Emmett A. *A Brief History of Physical Education*. Rev. ed. New York: A. S. Barnes, 1929.

Strutt, Joseph. *The Sports and Pastimes of the People of England*. London: William Tegg, 1850.

Van Dalen, Deobald B., and Bennett, Bruce L. *A World History of Physical Education*. 2d ed. Englewood Cliffs, N.J.: Prentice-Hall, 1971.

Vendien, C. Lynn, and Nixon, John E. *The World Today in Health, Physical Education and Recreation*. Englewood Cliffs, N.J.: Prentice-Hall, 1968.

von Hagen, Victor Wolfgang. *The Ancient Sun Kingdoms of the Americas*. Cleveland: World, 1961.

Chapter 3
Philosophical
Foundations

The unexamined life is not
worth living.

SOCRATES

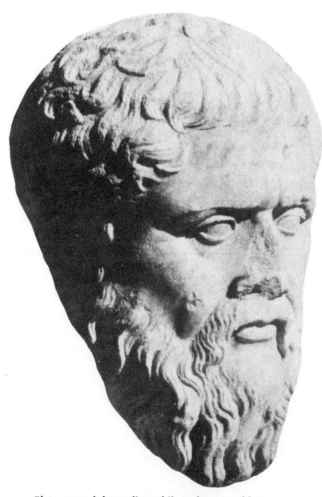

Plato, one of the earliest philosophers to address sport.

WHAT is the purpose of sport? What is the place of physical education in a hierarchy of curriculum matter? Do organized programs of competitive athletics contribute in a positive way to one's value system? Is it important for individuals to know themselves, to develop their personal identities? Are human beings basically motivated by what Frankl calls the "will to meaning?"[1] Can they be nurtured toward "defining their essence" through physical education and sport?

Thoughtful answers to these questions require something called philosophizing. Philosophy can be loosely defined as the love of wisdom, and the formal study of philosophy involves three main branches: metaphysics, the study of the nature of reality; epistemology, the study of the nature of knowing; and axiology, the study of values. Various schools or systems of philosophy (for example, pragmatism, realism, idealism, and existentialism) identify quite distinctive theories in each of these areas. Although it may not be necessary to embrace a particular system of philosophy, it is imperative to be consistent in one's beliefs and to base one's actions on them. Such consistency cannot evolve without heeding Socrates' dictum cited at the beginning of this chapter. Each person needs to make certain decisions about his or her goals and values. Unfortunately, perhaps, there is not a sports official to fire a gun to start one down the road of self-examination. The decision to initiate such activity must be made by individuals and they must follow through largely on their own. All kinds of people and all sorts of conditions can serve as a catalyst for the search, but the decision to act is a personal, extremely significant one.

THE BRANCHES OF PHILOSOPHY

A basic awareness of the main branches of philosophy—metaphysics, epistemology, and axiology—and what is entailed in each seems essential if one is to begin to understand the discipline of philosophy.

Metaphysics is concerned with the nature of reality, including ultimate reality, and to think metaphysically is to reflect on the most basic problems and questions of existence. It is perhaps only the rare, reflective person who truly questions the meaning and purpose of life. There appear to be at least two aspects of reality, the physical (matter) and the mental (mind). How can we make compatible two such diverse "realities"? For years we in physical education and sport have been arguing that there is no dichotomy between mind and body. On what basis can such an argument be founded? Attention to the study of metaphysics should help us formulate a tenable position.

Epistemology, the study of theories of knowledge, has as its central concern what it is that we can know. This is at once one of the most important and most difficult questions in philosophy. The theories regarding the source of knowledge range from empiricism (the view that all knowledge comes from sense data), to rationalism (the view that reason must organize sense experience if it is to be meaningful), to intuition (the view that there is a total response to a total situation which supplements both reason and the senses). If there is a totality of body and mind, then how we come to know has great import in physical education. Can we come to know with our bodies? If so, do we need to pay greater attention to pedagogical behavior so that such knowledge can be nurtured?

Axiology, the study of values, is essential if we are to have a comprehensive view of humanity and the world. Everyone has standards, convictions, loyalties, and the like, but not everyone has examined his or her value spectrum for consistency. One of the fundamental questions in axiology is whether value judgments express feelings or knowledge, and various theories subscribe to one or the other of these positions. Regardless of the theory, it would seem to be important for us to discover and nurture the genuine values of life. Axiology can be divided into two main areas, ethics and aesthetics, and each of these is of extreme worth in a unified view of physical education and sport. *Ethics,* the study of right and wrong, or morality, ought to be of central concern to us all if we are to rise above instinctual, animal-like behavior. Especially in sport, perhaps, the question of values and disvalues are or ought to be paramount. On every hand one sees the dehumanization and manipulation of athletes. Can such practices be condoned for any reason? It would seem that thoughtful attention to such questions must be addressed if organized athletics are to survive. *Aesthetics,* the study of the beautiful, is likewise essential in the discipline of physical education if we believe that human movement can be beautiful, that the body in motion can be a true aesthetic object, and that one can experience the "aesthetic moment" in physical activity. There are, of course, many and divergent aesthetic theories; some of them at least partially support the above contentions while others reject them entirely. The physical educator ought to be more knowledgeable about them before making aesthetic claims for physical activity which are perhaps unwarranted.

TYPES OF PHILOSOPHIC THINKING AND RESEARCH

The field of philosophy typically exhibits three types of thinking and research. The first type is *speculative,* in which inferences are made based on large amounts of data or factual information. Take, for example, the observation that there is increasing evidence of organized gambling at all levels of sport. Upon speculation, can this fact be used to justify the contention that there is a moral decline in sport? The second type is *analytic,* in which an attempt is made to analyze concepts, relation-

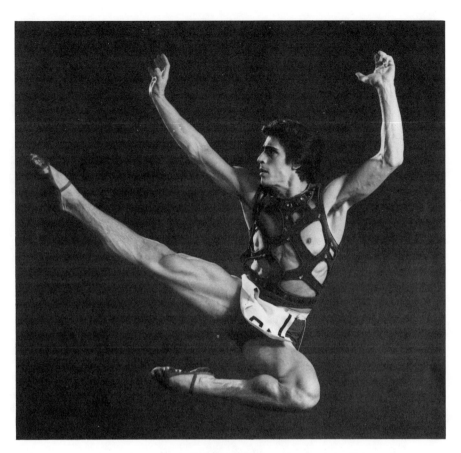

The athlete as artist (Edward Villella, New York City Ballet)
(Photograph by Martha Swope)

ships, component parts, and even words and idioms. Analytic philosophy is concerned especially with logic, language, and concepts. An example is the question whether physical education can truly be considered an academic discipline. The third type is *critical* or *normative,* in which value judgments are made and norms or standards are proposed. For example, ought a program of physical education be required of all pupils in our schools?

In addition to the above, *phenomenological* research has blossomed in recent years and, according to many physical education scholars, it seems to offer the best possible avenue for investigating the *essence* of physical activity and how such essence helps the individual to define his or her self. Edmund Husserl, the father of phenomenology, called for a "return to the things themselves;" that is, a return to unadulterated phenomena. Husserl's methodology is understood only with great difficulty; however, the phenomenology of such existential philosophers as Jean-Paul Sartre and Maurice Merleau-Ponty seems more germane and especially applicable to physical education and sport. Phenomenologists aim

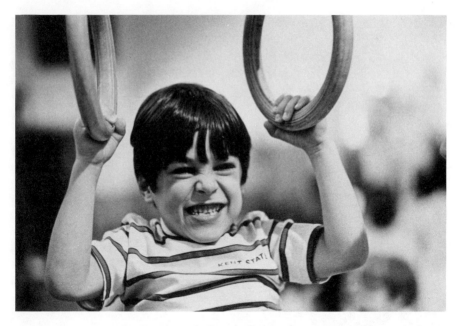

The joy of effort

to explore the nature of consciousness in order to reveal the meaning of existence and, at least for Sartre and Merleau-Ponty, the body plays a significant role in bestowing essence on existence.

INTERRELATIONSHIP OF PHILOSOPHY AND PHYSICAL EDUCATION

If physical education is defined as the art and science of human movement and if philosophy is defined as the love of wisdom, can these two disciplines interrelate for mutual benefit? Historically, philosophy is referred to as the "Queen of the Sciences." As such, philosophy nurtured the knowledge in all fields which subsequently appeared. Whereas science is concerned with the acquisition of detailed facts (knowledge), philosophy is concerned with the critical examination of those facts as well as with the relationship among sets of facts within and among different disciplines (wisdom). William James, a Pragmatist, once noted that philosophy deals with a "peculiarly stubborn effort to think clearly." Thus it is a process of reasoned reflection which uses logic as its chief tool and which aims toward an understanding of humanity, of the universe, and of their relationships. It appears obvious that the knowledge generated by and through scientific endeavor is of extreme import to the philosopher; often the philosopher is also a scientist and the scientist a philosopher. The philosopher and the scientist who work within the discipline of physical education must work closely together if each arm of the discipline is to benefit. The problem of anabolic steroids is but one isolated example of a concern that ought to be mutual. The scientific researcher in physical education can arrive at facts about whether or not the use of anabolic steroids can build muscle mass and improve motor performance. Assuming affirmative answers, the question yet remains whether it is ethical for athletes to use such ergogenic aids. The answer falls within the purview of the philosopher in physical education and sport.

Movement as an art form deals primarily with expression, communication, form, and beauty. Is there anything in physical education which can properly be called an art form? Perhaps if some physical educators were to embark upon a serious study of aesthetics answers which are more than mere prejudicial statements could be at least tentatively proffered. We in physical education almost invariably think of gymnastics as art, but is it? Does the fact that specific skills must be included in a routine and must be performed in a certain way in order to earn a high mark from the judges negate creativity and thus art?

The founding of the Philosophic Society for the Study of Sport in 1972 is evidence of the growing interest in questions surrounding our engagement in physical activity. Philosophers of all kinds, including education and physical education, comprise the membership of this international society which sponsors an annual conference and also publishes the *Journal of the Philosophy of Sport*. Further evidence of interest can be seen in the increasing number of books, articles, and research papers published concerning philosophy of sport.[2]

If philosophy is the love of wisdom and if wisdom is a culmination of knowledge and understanding, then let us hope that the discipline of physical education will begin to rely more heavily on philosophic thinking in order to guide it toward a potential development that permits a life- and world-view based on a holistic concept of a thinking, feeling, and moving individual.

STUDENT PROJECTS

1. Delve into *Doctoral Dissertation Abstracts* and the *University of Oregon H.P.E.R. Microfilm Publications Bulletin* for papers done in the general area of philosophy of physical education and sport. Make a list of them and try to decide what type of philosophic thinking was involved.

2. Physical educators often cite Plato as an advocate of their discipline. What did Plato really say about the body?

3. Have you ever been motivated in a physical education class to reflect, other than kinesthetically, about how your body "feels" when in motion? How might a physical education teacher motivate such reflection?

4. Survey a group of coaches and prospective coaches about what they consider to be the purpose of sport.

5. As a start down the path of self-examination, write a short paper entitled, "This I Believe," in which you reflect on several diverse topics, such as the value of education, your relationship with a Supreme Being, parenthood, and the joy of effort in sport.

GLOSSARY OF TERMS

Philosophy   The love of wisdom.

Metaphysics   The study of the nature of reality.

Epistemology   The study of theories of knowledge.

Axiology   The study of values.

Ethics   The study of right and wrong or morality.

Aesthetics   The study of the beautiful.

REFERENCES

1. V. E. Frankl, "The Alienation and Identity of Man in Sport," *Sport in the Modern World—Chances and Problems* (Berlin: Springer-Verlag, 1973).

2. For example, see Michael Novak's *The Joy of Sport*, Paul Weiss' *Sport: A Philosophic Inquiry*, Robert Osterhoudt's *The Philosophy of Sport*, and a recent (Fall 1976) issue of *Philosophy Today* devoted almost exclusively to sport.

SELECTED READINGS

"Athletics and Education, Are They Compatible?" *Phi Delta Kappan,* LVI:2 (October 1974). Entire Issue.

Coutts, Curtis A. "Freedom in Sport." *Quest* **10** (May 1968).

Gerber, Ellen. "Identity, Relation and Sport." *Quest* **8** (May 1967).

Gerber, Ellen, ed. *Sport and the Body.* Philadelphia: Lea & Febiger, 1972.

Kleinman, Seymour. "Toward a Non-Theory of Sport." *Quest* **10** (May 1968).

Leonard, George. *The Ultimate Athlete.* New York: Viking, 1974.

Michener, James A. *Sports in America.* New York: Random House, 1976.

Novak, Michael. *The Joy of Sports.* New York: Basic Books, 1976.

Osterhoudt, Robert, ed. *The Philosophy of Sport.* Springfield, Ill.: Charles C Thomas, 1973.

"Perspectives on the Philosophy of Sport." *The Scientific View of Sport*. Berlin: Springer-Verlag, 1972.

"Sport and Play—Philosophical Interpretations" and "The Alienation and Identity of Man in Sport." In *Sport in the Modern World—Chances and Problems*. Berlin: Springer-Verlag, 1973.

VanderZwaag, Harold. *Toward a Philosophy of Sport*. Reading, Mass.: Addison-Wesley, 1972.

Weiss, Paul. *Sport: A Philosophic Inquiry*. Carbondale: Southern Illinois University Press, 1969.

Chapter 4 Biomechanical Foundations

The laws of physics are the decrees of Fate.

ALFRED NORTH WHITEHEAD

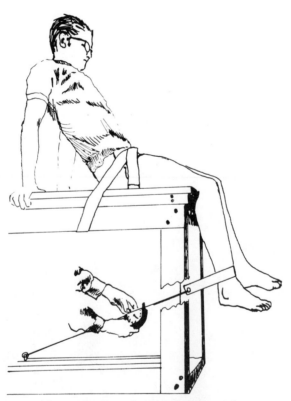

A measurement of extensor torque at the knee joint using a cable tensiometer.

THE NEXT three chapters of this text are devoted to the foundations of physical education, as derived from the areas of biomechanics, anatomy, physiology, and the behavioral sciences of sociology and psychology. Physical education is an applied science which finds its basic principles within these scientific areas. The human being as a moving, living body obeys the scientific laws of the universe. With adequate knowledge of scientific truths and the application of them to our efforts, we can move more efficiently and propel objects to greater height and distances with accuracy.

For many years the bulk of all research in physical education was centered either in curriculum or in teaching and coaching methods. To fill the need for additional knowledge about the effects of exercise or activity on the human body, the area of exercise physiology developed with its own laboratories and research personnel. Similarly, when more knowledge was needed on how the body moved, both kinesiological and myographic laboratories came into being. More recently, investigation by the profession in the area of motor learning has encompassed both the sociological and the physical impact of physical activity on humans. Research and research facilities in this area are now an integral part of many departments, and the results are being presented in the research sections of many professional meetings.

In this chapter the authors reviewed those laws of physics which have special meaning to people or the materials we use in our physical activities. Examples from exercise and sports illustrate how adherence to the physical laws can help in both participation and teaching.

Basically, the material is set forth by means of guiding principles for the professional physical educator. A definition of the term "principle" should clarify its use in this context. As used in the field, *principles of physical education are guides to behavior based on truth as determined by the scientific and philosophical knowledge of the times.* When science discovers new truths and philosophic concepts change, or when new philosophies evolve, the underlying principles of the discipline also change.

BIOMECHANICAL SCIENCES—GENERAL COMMENTS

All objects on earth are responsive to the laws of the physical world, whether they are in motion or at complete rest. These laws apply to the body, its movements, and the objects it manipulates. Since all physical activity revolves around human movement, a serious student should understand the internal and external forces which are constantly brought into play. The science of movement stems from the disciplines of biology and physics.

Many physical activities are concerned with the propulsion of objects by lifting, throwing, pushing, or striking. Although most participants operate on the level of kinesthesis (the way the activity feels), physical education teachers and coaches should have a working knowledge of the biomechanical principles involved. The study of kinematics (quantitative description of motion) enables the students to determine the orientation as the object moves. They are then able to relate the principles to the various activities and to evaluate instruction and performance in the light of this knowledge. They may violate one of the principles to achieve a greater adherence to another. For example, one might sacrifice stability to increase forward movement, knowing what that decision will cost.

Entire textbooks have been written about the physical and mechanical principles as they apply to a single sports activity. Therefore the examples of physical principles chosen are such that they apply to most sports, with specific reference to selected ones for purposes of clarification and explanation. The mechanics of physical activity is a relatively new and fertile field for study and research.

INTERNAL FORCES OF HUMAN MOVEMENT

The body moves and applies force to objects by contracting muscles (force) which act across joints (axes) by means of a system of levers (bones). When a stimulus reaches a muscle through a motor nerve impulse, biological energy is converted to mechanical movement. The intensity of the movement depends on the number of muscle fibers stimulated.

The levers in the body follow the classification used in the external physical world. By definition, a lever is a simple machine which facilitates work by means of a fixed fulcrum and a rigid body or arm. The classifications are made according to the location of the axis (fulcrum) in relation to the two forces, effort and resistance. In a first-class lever, the fulcrum (A) is located between the resistance (R) and the effort (E), as illustrated in Fig. 4.1. Common examples of this type of lever are crowbars, scissors, pliers, balances (scales), and seesaws. The extension of the arm at the elbow by the triceps and the extension of the foot at the ankle when not bearing weight are examples within the body. A pole vaulter

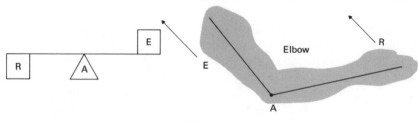

FIGURE 4.1

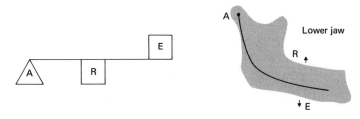

FIGURE 4.2

approaching with the pole in the "carry" position is an example of this lever. In terms of work done by any effort, this type of lever is most efficient.

In the second-class lever, the resistance, or weight, is located between the fulcrum and the effort, or force (Fig. 4.2). Examples of this type are a wheelbarrow, a nutcracker, and a paper trimmer. There are very few examples of this type of lever in the body but one is the lower jaw. Another occurs in running when the runner pushes off the toes.

Most levers of the human body are of the third class, in which the effort is located between the fulcrum and the resistance (Fig. 4.3). Shovels, sugar tongs, and grass shears are examples of third-class levers. Two examples in the human body are the flexions of the lower arm and lower leg. In the case of the arm, as in Fig. 4.3, the biceps attaches in the forearm on the radius. This lever lends itself to the development of speed of movement, because the resistance arm is longer than the force arm. Some joints act as more than one class of lever; the elbow may be used as an example of all three.

In all three lever types, a state of balance or equilibrium is determined by the formula,

$$\text{Force} \times \text{Force arm} = \text{Resistance} \times \text{Resistance arm.}$$

Movement results from an increase in either force or resistance or from the shortening or lengthening of either of the two arms. The distance from the axis to the point of effort is the effort (force) arm, while the distance from the axis to the point of resistance is the resistance arm. In the first-class lever, a great resistance can be overcome with little force by lengthening the force arm. In the human body, one may obtain

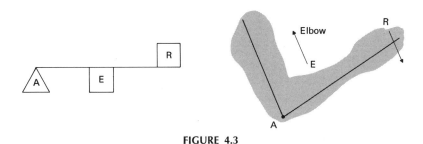

FIGURE 4.3

speed of movement by using a force on a resistance with a long resistance arm. Implements such as rackets, paddles, oars, and bats increase the length of the lever arms.

In most movements of the body, a number of levers come into action simultaneously or in sequence. This fact may require the stabilizing of other parts of the body, as occurs in heavy weight lifting.

CENTER OF GRAVITY

For a definition of gravity or gravitation, Sir Isaac Newton's principle should suffice. He stated that between any two objects in the world there exists a mutual force of attraction that is directly proportional to the product of the masses of the objects and inversely proportional to the square of their distances apart. Since the earth has such an enormous mass, the attraction to it is greater than between two smaller objects. For example, if one held two baseballs at arm's length and released them, the attraction between them would be negligible in comparison with the attraction of each to the mass of the earth (Fig. 4.4). The baseballs would fall to earth; thus the weight of an object is determined by this gravitational pull of the earth. An object is attracted to earth with the acceleration of 32 feet per second for each second of fall (wind resistance discounted).

In all physical activities these principles apply. Objects propelled in sports are affected in their flight, as is the body when it swings, hangs, and moves. The center of gravity of a body is the point at which its whole weight can be brought into balance. In a simple symmetrical object like a ball, the center of gravity is usually the literal center. In an irregularly shaped object like the human body or a baseball bat, it may be more difficult to determine. The human body moves and its parts change their relationships to one another; with such changes there is a change in the center of gravity. For example, the raising of the arms over the head elevates the center of gravity by several centimeters.

In both equilibrium and motion, the center of gravity plays an important role. The stable position of the defensive football lineman or of the wrestler differs from that of a trackman on the starting blocks. The body is balanced when the center of gravity is above the base of support.

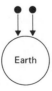

FIGURE 4.4

That result can be achieved by simply spreading the feet apart, but if one carries the adjustment to extremes, one becomes so stable one cannot move. The larger base gives a greater balance in that the center of gravity is kept within the base. The center of gravity in the human body may vary from person to person according to body build and sex. The center of gravity of the male is usually higher than that of the female. Movements during walking, running, and kicking will raise, lower, or change the lateral position of the center of gravity. Since the center of gravity may fall either within or without the body, balance depends upon the ability to change the position of the center of gravity to meet the movement requirements of the sport.

In running events the center of gravity is kept in front of the base of support to give a pulling effect. In tumbling and diving a high center of gravity helps the performer in rotary movements. The offensive backs in football use a stance that is different from that of the defensive lineman. The degree of stability necessary for these positions varies; hence the center of gravity of the players is altered.

MOTION

In 1687 Sir Isaac Newton wrote a treatise on motion which became the basis of modern mechanics. Newton propounded three simple basic laws of motion, which are equally applicable today with a few minor exceptions that are far beyond the scope of this text.

Newton's first law: Every body (object) persists in a state of rest or of uniform motion in a straight line unless compelled by external forces to change that state.

This law of motion deals with the overcoming of the tendency of rest or, in physical terms, inertia. Let us examine some examples from activity. In track or baseball the runner makes better time from a running start than from a stationary one. Baseball runners must tag up (touch base) before advancing on a fly ball. It would be to the runner's advantage to approach the base from the far side and time his or her touch with the catch. Some years ago a rule was placed in the books to prohibit this approach. A quarter miler achieves better time from a flying start, as in a relay, than from a dead start. Other examples of this principle are the windup of the pitcher or the push-off in bowling, which puts the ball in motion to overcome the inertia of twelve to sixteen pounds at rest and results in a greater ball speed and smoother delivery. Another example of the impact of Newton's first law is that a baseball rolls much farther or faster on the new synthetic surfaces and may change the strategy of the game in such instances where the infield must play deeper or the bunt travels faster.

An illustration of persistence in motion in a straight line is the tendency of base runners or trackrunners to swing wide in making their turns;

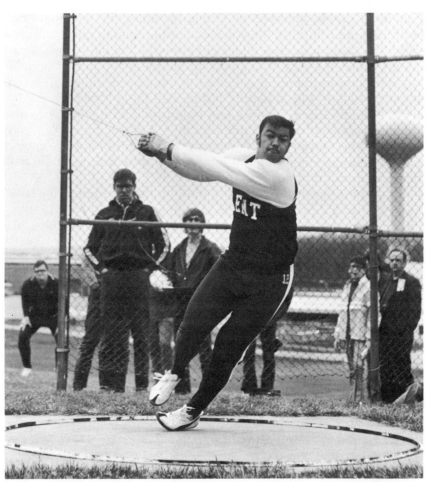

Hammer thrower pulls inward as a counter-balance to keep hammer from flying off in a straight line or tangent. Photo courtesy of Kent State University Department of Intercollegiate Athletics.

they must apply force to the base, ground, or track to change this tendency. Base runners slide into the base to avoid overrunning it, since the body persists in a state of motion. Hammer throwers have to pull inward to prevent the hammer from flying off at a tangent.

Newton's second law: When a body (object is acted upon by a force, its resultant acceleration (change of speed) is proportional to the force and inversely proportional to the mass.

One of the forces which must be contended with in activity is gravity. This constant force of 32 feet per second/per second must be considered in such events as the high jump, the pole vault, and throwing. The golfer must consider the force necessary to propel the ball to the green by changing the club or the speed of the swing. The basketball player must learn the force necessary to reach the basket from different ranges within the shooting area.

Newton's third law: For every force or action there is an equal and opposite reaction.

In physical activity and sports, this particular law of motion plays a major role. The act of moving one's body on air, land, and water depends on it. When sprinters push against the surface of the track, the reaction propels them forward. When swimmers press against the water, the reaction propels them in the opposite direction. The force exerted on the floor elevates the body in a push-up. Finally, in all striking activities, action and reaction occur. When two such objects as a racket and a ball meet, there is a reaction in both. This phenomenon will be explored more fully in the next few sections.

Motion in athletics may be described in terms of speed or velocity, which is simply a function of distance and time. A factor which is equally important in sports, however, is the ability to accelerate. Acceleration is defined as the rate of change in velocity in a set period of time. Acceleration may be either positive or negative, and both are equally important in sport. Positive acceleration is typified by a standing start, such as a start in track or a sudden burst of speed of a half-back finding an opening in the line. Negative acceleration is the necessary slowing down to perform in sports, as when the base runner slides to prevent over-running the base and the basketball dribbler slows down to change direction.

CONSERVATION OF MOMENTUM

In a collision between two objects, whatever momentum is gained by one object has been lost by the other, and the momentum of the whole system remains the same. This principle may be shown by the formula

$$MV + M'V' = MU + M'U',$$

where M represents the mass of the first object, V represents its velocity before the collision, and M' and V' represent respectively the weight and velocity of the second object. After the collision, U and U' represent the new velocities of the first and second objects, respectively. In a specific example, a pitched baseball with a mass of 5 oz is traveling at 90 mph and strikes a 32 oz bat traveling at 90 mph. If the speed of the bat is reduced to 80 mph, the hit ball will travel at 154 mph. Transferring these values to the formula above, we have

$$(5)(90) + 32(90) = (5)(x) + 32(80),$$

and solving for x gives us the speed of 154 mph for the hit ball.

The swing of the striking end of the bat is the most important factor. Within limits, a lighter bat permits the average player to develop this

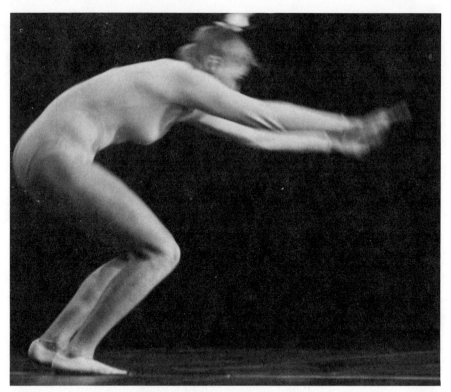

Sprinters coming out of the blocks and gymnasts doing flips and rolls are but two examples of Newton's "Action-Reaction Law." Photos courtesy of Kent State University Department of Intercollegiate Athletics.

speed without a significant loss in the total sum of forces. The batter's stride, pivot, and wrist action all contribute to the speed of the striking portion of the bat. In a similar problem, a golf ball sitting on a tee by a driver. The entire sum of the momentum gained by both driver and ball must be supplied by the driver, since the golf ball is at rest at the start, and therefore the mass of the golf ball is multiplied by zero velocity. As in the baseball example, the club head speed is the dominating factor if we assume that all the other conditions remain stable. The same principle holds true for a ball dropped on a hard-surface floor of an infinite mass. Theoretically, the ball will rebound to a height from which it falls; however, the formula above requires the following conditions: (1) the objects meet at the center of gravity

$$q \qquad \rightarrow \!\! \circ\!\!\circ \!\! \leftarrow$$

or, as expressed in sports, "on the button"; (2) the objects travel without rotation or spin; (3) there is no heat or sound energy lost; and (4) the objects have a perfect "coefficient of restitution," or elasticity. The loss

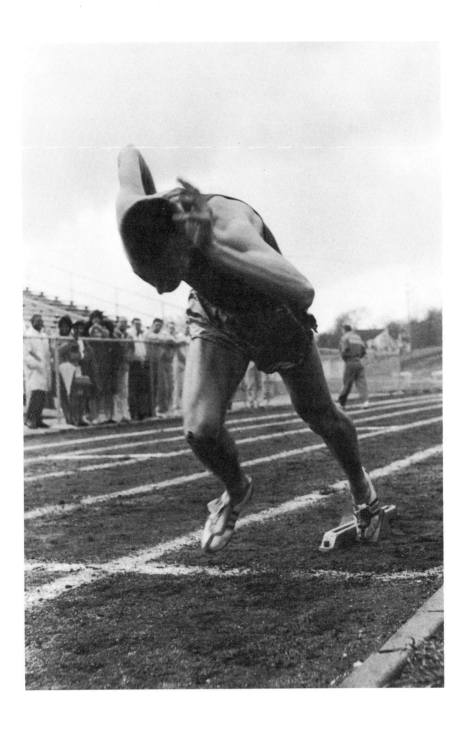

of speed is explained by these four factors since the principle of conservation of energy holds that *energy cannot be manufactured or destroyed; it can only be directed in its flow or transformed.*

COEFFICIENT OF RESTITUTION

One of the conditions cited for the perfect conservation of momentum was that of a perfect "coefficient of restitution." This term simply means that the object can return to its original shape rapidly after being compressed by a blow. This capability varies in accordance with differences in materials and methods used in the construction of the objects. Golf balls especially vary in this quality. Cheaper balls are usually less elastic, in addition to having other undesirable features, such as low resistance to cuts and less whiteness of cover. A ball filled with air is easily compressed, but it returns to its original shape more slowly than does a solid ball of elastic material. A simple test can demonstrate this principle. With a yardstick held perpendicular to a hard, smooth surface, have several balls dropped a distance of one yard to the surface, and record the heights of the rebounds. For each ball the percentage of return, which shows the amount of elasticity, is its "coefficient of restitution." The readings could vary from 0 to a perfect coefficient of 1 (Fig. 4.5).

For obtaining an exact coefficient of restitution, we have the formula[1]

$$e = \frac{hb}{hd},$$

where e is the coefficient of elasticity, *hb* is the height of the bounce, and *hd* is the height of the drop.

The elastic quality of a ball may be altered by a change in temperature. Handballs are often placed in hot water prior to use to make them livelier. In recent years a number of baseball managers have been

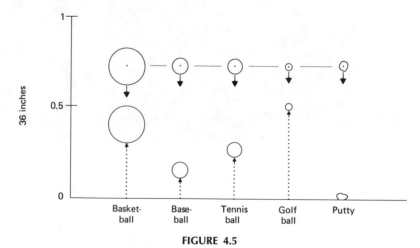

FIGURE 4.5

accused of keeping baseballs under refrigeration when playing teams of superior hitting abilities. Some differences can be expected in balls of the same materials and workmanship, and such differences tend to be more noticeable when there is a loss of elasticity due to use and aging.

ROTATION OR SPIN

Much of the success of a participant in games involving balls (especially round ones) is due to his or her ability to impart the proper amount of rotation or spin in the direction desired. The baseball pitcher, the golfer, the handball player, the tennis player, and the bowler have much in common in that the rotation of the manipulated object may be the key to success. A "moving" fastball or one that leaves its initial line of flight is harder to hit than one that travels faster but straighter.

What are the physical laws of rotation and spin, and how do they function? A simplified explanation is that when a struck or thrown ball is spinning, the side that turns into the air wall (or solid material) meets with increased resistance, whereas the side turning away from the direction of flight meets less resistance and therefore tends to accelerate. This combination of circumstances causes the ball to rise, fall, hook, or slice. When a backspin is imparted to it, a ball will tend to rise and, on striking a surface, turn toward the striker or thrower. This explains both the "hop" (rise) on a fastball, and the backspin on a golf ball that is properly hit to the green (Fig. 4.6). The ball follows the path of least resistance, as shown in Fig. 4.7. The ball is impeded in its turn in toward the surface at point A but free to turn at point B.

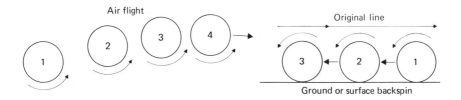

FIGURE 4.6

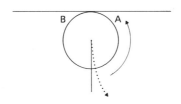

FIGURE 4.7

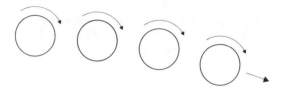

FIGURE 4.8

If top spin is imparted to it, a ball will drop faster, because of the factors described above, but it will roll away from the thrower or striker (Fig. 4.8). The rebound will be harder and faster. Tennis and table tennis players use top spin to cause the ball to strike in a prescribed area and rebound rapidly. In baseball the "sinker" or "drop" ball pitcher uses this technique.

A clockwise rotation imparted to a ball will cause the ball to move toward the thrower's or striker's right (Fig. 4.9). The right-handed player will make the bowling ball fade, slice the golf ball, and throw an in-curve in baseball. In striking games there is usually some loss of distance because of clockwise rotation.

A counterclockwise rotation imparted to a ball by a right-handed striker or thrower moves the ball to the left of the original line of flight (Fig. 4.10). This results in an out-curve for the pitcher and a hook for the bowler or golfer.

Other objects in sports have special problems. When a football is kicked (punted) or thrown, it is rotated in order to stabilize it and to reduce the wind resistance. The nose is elevated or depressed, depending on the distance desired or the wind conditions. The discus and the javelin have special problems of aerodynamics because of their size

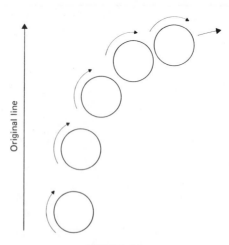

FIGURE 4.9

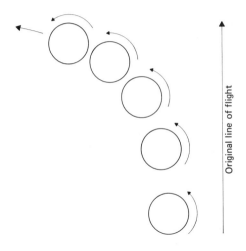

Original line of flight

FIGURE 4.10

and shape. These problems and others are studied in advanced courses in the mechanics of physical activities.

The trajectory of any body is resultant of two actions, e.g., the forward and upward velocity of that body. As described in the early section on gravity, whenever anybody (athlete or object) loses contact with the ground the forces of gravity act upon that body and it begins to fall. Whenever a discus is thrown or a golf ball struck, if we disregard wind resistance, the resultant of the two forces (gravity and forward velocity) determines how far these objects will travel. Ordinarily the optimum angle of the trajectory is 45 degress; however, air resistance and any differential between point of release and landing are factors. Hitting a golf ball from a high tee to a much lower green is an example of this exception. This principle, together with the aerodynamics of such sports objects as the javelin and discus, are the subject of much research.

SUMMARY

Teachers and coaches must have an understanding of simple mechanics since the human body moves within the framework of these universal laws. Furthermore, the implements used in sports can be handled more efficiently if both player and coach have an understanding of the basic principles involved. Although scientific principles are sometimes defied with some degree of success, the instructor should have an understanding of what is lost or gained by such defiance.

When a baseball player, golfer, or tennis player selects a longer or heavier bat, club, or racquet, he or she should be aware of the consequences of the choice. If a player has a choice between a stiff shaft and a flexible one, the teacher should point out the advantages and disadvantages of each. It is not enough for the teacher or coach to instruct student players in how to perform; they must also know why they should perform in that way.

Finally, bodily injuries may occur when mechanical principles are ignored or insufficiently understood. The acts of standing and walking, if done improperly, may result in weak and fallen arches. Improper lifting may cause a painful back condition. Throwing curve balls (especially the screwball) may cause permanent damage to young baseball players who are allowed to throw an excessive number of them.

STUDENT PROJECTS

1. Bring to class various balls that are normally used in different sports. Impart spin to them on the floor and on the desk tops. Observe the path taken by a ball after it strikes an obstruction, such as a wall.
2. Drop a number of balls of different types from the same level and observe the height of the rebound. Estimate the coefficients of restitution.

GLOSSARY OF TERMS

Principles Guides to behavior based on truth as determined by the scientific and philosophical knowledge of the times.

Kinesiology The study of human motion.

Center of gravity The point at which the whole weight of a body can be brought into balance.

Conservation of momentum The principle that total momentum remains the same in a collision bewteen two objects. Whatever momentum is gained by one object has been lost by the other.

Coefficient of restitution The rate at which an object returns to its original shape after being compressed by a blow.

Kinematics Quantitative description of motion.

REFERENCES

1. John W. Bunn, *Scientific Principles of Coaching* (New York: Prentice-Hall, 1955), pp. 65–66.

SELECTED READINGS

Broer, Marian R. *Efficiency of Human Movement*. 3d ed. Philadelphia: W. B. Saunders, 1973.

Bunn, John W. *Scientific Principles of Coaching.* New York: Prentice-Hall, 1955.

Constant, F. Woodbridge. *Fundamental Principles of Physics.* Reading, Mass.: Addison-Wesley, 1967.

Dyson, Geoffrey H. G. *The Mechanics of Athletics.* 4th ed. London: University of London Press, 1967.

Groves, Richard, and Camaoine, David N. *Concepts in Kinesiology.* Philadelphia: W. B. Saunders, 1975.

Hay, James G. *The Biomechanics of Sports Techniques.* Englewood Cliffs, N.J.: Prentice-Hall, 1973.

Read, Albert J. *Physics: A Descriptive Analysis.* Reading, Mass.: Addison-Wesley, 1970.

Trickner, R. A. R., and Trickner, B. J. K. *The Science of Movement.* New York: American Elsevier, 1967.

Wickstrom, Ralph L. *Fundamental Motor Patterns.* Philadelphia: Lea & Febiger, 1970, pp. 16–19.

Williams, Marian, and Lessner, Herbert R. *Biomechanics of Human Motion.* Philadelphia: W. B. Saunders, 1962, pp. 111–128.

Chapter 5
Anatomical
and
Physiological
Foundations

Health is the vital principle
of bliss,
And exercise, of health.

JAMES THOMSON

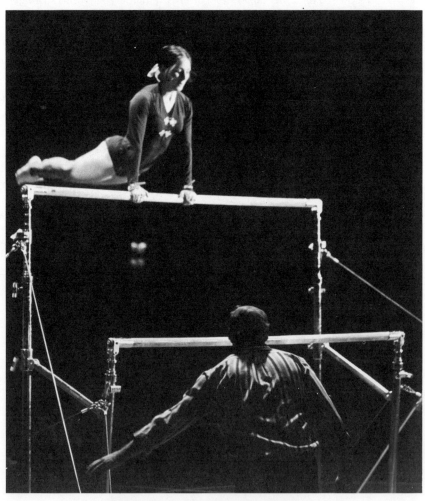

**Skillful movement involves a knowledge of
anatomical and physiological principles.**

HOW the body is structured (anatomy) and how it functions (physiology) determine to a great degree how a person performs physical activities, including athletic sports. Some capacities of a given individual are established at conception by the genetic characteristics inherited from parents. Others can be changed by conditioning the systems of the body to perform the desired activities at optimum levels. The purpose of this chapter is to examine some general anatomical and physiological principles and the practical application of these principles in specific situations. Study in depth in these areas is essential for all teachers of physical education, who will find the opportunity for such study in most curricula of teacher preparation institutions offering a major program.

ANATOMICAL PRINCIPLES

The body type (build) of an individual has an important influence on physical performance

There are a number of ways of determining body types (somatotyping), from that of Sheldon, who classified three basic body types, to that of Wetzel, who devised nine channels. There are very few pure body types. Most individuals have characteristics from two of Sheldon's types, with occasionally a few from the third. The three principal body types as described by Sheldon follow.

Endomorphic. Persons with endomorphic characteristics are usually short, soft in appearance, and rounded in contour. Their heads are large and rounded, their necks are short and thick, their shoulders are rounded, their chests are barrel-shaped, and their abdomens larger than their chests. Their arms and legs are short and thick, and they have short, pudgy fingers and toes.

Mesomorphic. Persons with mesomorphic characteristics are muscular, of medium height, and square or triangular in appearance. Their heads are average with square features, their necks are average in length but muscular, and their shoulders are wide and square. Their chests are broad and elliptical, their buttocks and hips are small, their arms and legs are average in length but muscular in outline, and their hands and feet are average in size.

Ectomorphic. Persons with ectomorphic characteristics are usually tall, thin, and sharp-featured. Their heads are small, their features sharp, and they have long, thin necks. Their shoulders are narrow and thin, their chests are narrow, and they have long trunks. Their arms and legs are long and thin, and their hands and feet are large.

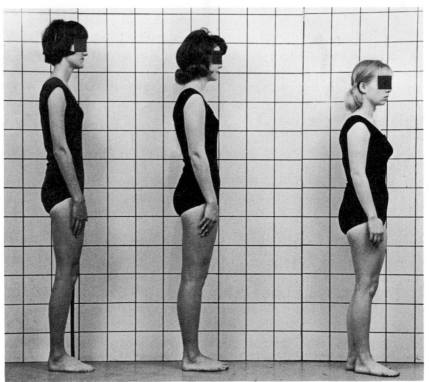

Examples of different body types. Photo courtesy of Department of Physical Education, Kent State University.

The average female, in comparison with the average male, tends toward the endomorphic type. Several subprinciples involving this comparison follow.

1. *The carrying angle (arm angle)* is greater in the female than in the male. As illustrated in Fig. 5.1, the narrowness of the shoulders of the female and the width of the pelvic girdle contribute to this difference, which expresses itself in the fact that girls carry books at the breast level, whereas boys carry them at the extended arm position. Another example of the effect of the carrying angle is suggested by the off-center placement of the handle in modern luggage in order to give a better mechanical advantage. Note, however, that the difference in carrying angle is not the principal reason that girls throw differently than boys; the reason is more likely to be that they were not given proper instruction during their formative years.

2. *The oblique leg line is greater in the female than the male.* The female's broader pelvic girdle after adolescence gives her femur a marked obliquity compared with that of the male. As the schematic view of Fig. 5.2 indicates, the mechanical advantage remains with the male. The greater obliquity produces side sway and oscillation; the latter in turn

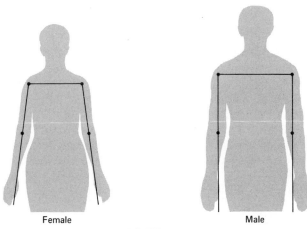

Female   Male

FIGURE 5.1

reduces forward speed and resembles the side sway produced by cross-body arm action in running. Fashion models exaggerate this movement when they walk by placing one foot before the other.

This principle is illustrated by the excellent girl runners who tend to have the body build depicted in the diagram on the right. They have very little side sway and therefore greater forward speed.

3. *The pelvis of the female is wider and more shallow than that of the male.* Although the wider pelvis of the female is important for child-bearing, the greater prominence of the hips works to her disadvantage in the preceding two subprinciples. Female pelvises are not all of the same shape, however, and some women have the narrow, deep pelvis of the male, which may complicate the delivery of their children. In all areas of bodily differences specified in these three subprinciples, there may be variations. The female may have the structure described as male,

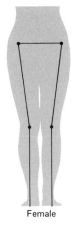 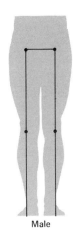

Female   Male

FIGURE 5.2

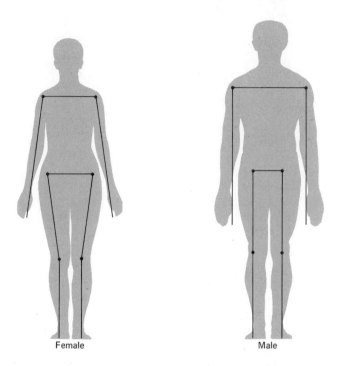

Female   Male

FIG. 5.3 A composite schematic view of the typical male and female figures, depicting the differences in arm angle, shoulder width, and pelvic width, as well as the obliquity of the femur.

whereas some males have wide hips, narrow shoulders, and lower centers of gravity, all of which are normally associated with the female. Such males may lose the mechanical advantage of forward running speed but gain in increased balance. The schematic view shown in Fig. 5.3, which combines Figs. 5.1 and 5.2, suggests the reason for the female's lower center of gravity as compared with that of the male. The advantages of both high and low centers of gravity were discussed in Chapter 4.

In summary, it may be stated that the two extremes in body types have often been maligned by physical educators and coaches; when they stress getting in "shape," they mean the shape of the ideal mesomorph. It should be kept in mind that the body type of an individual sets limits on the changes that can be made in the body by diet or activity. No amount of exercise would change a St. Bernard into a terrier, and no endomorph will become an ectomorph. He or she may, however, become a slimmer endomorph.

The endomorphic body types are often found among the football tackles and guards and in the weight events in track and field. Ectomorphs often dominate the long-distance running events, and they usually fill the center and forward positions in basketball. A low center of gravity is advantageous to a football fullback, whereas a high center of gravity helps a sprinter, because the body is thrust forward, thus creating a pulling effect. Clearly there are advantages and disadvantages in all body types.

PHYSIOLOGICAL PRINCIPLES

The environmental temperature has an effect on physical performance

When the environmental temperature rises above 80°F, body metabolism also rises. The number of respirations per minute increases by five or six with each rise of 1.8°F in rectal temperature. There is a rapid increase in pulse rate. There is a decrement in working capacity at 90°F from that at 70°F. In essence, extreme heat has the effect of detraining on an individual.

The human body can become acclimatized to heat. The period from the first exposure to the point at which acclimatization is well developed averages from five to eight days. The adjustment is less difficult if there is good physical conditioning, but it can be retarded by low salt and water intakes. Both water and salt should be available to the participant, but they should be used with care. For example, acclimatization is not improved by a higher than adequate salt intake. Acclimatization to heat is partially retained for several weeks and with occasional exposure can be extended for months.

The application of this principle is important in early football seasons, when heat stress tends to be a threat. Some states have forbidden the use of protective equipment for the first few days of practice for high school football players because it retards heat loss. At the college level, individual conferences have invoked a similar rule. Teams going to a hot climate to play (bowl games, for example) often arrive a week or two in advance of games in order to become acclimatized.

A cold environment also affects performance. Players do not receive enough benefits from warm-up. Furthermore, players on the bench and fans in the bleachers tighten their muscles in a cold environment. After a long period, these muscles are as fatigued as they would be if they had been used. The act of shivering is also fatiguing.

Water ingestion does not impede physical performance

As a result of heat-stress studies, there has been a decided reversal in the use of water during periods of vigorous physical performance. Whereas it was once common practice to forbid the use of water even in heat stress, water (or other liquids) is now made readily available, and participants are urged to replace lost fluids.

Since water makes up about seventy-five percent of muscle mass and salt another five percent, and since the composition of blood is eighty percent water, losses during heavy exercise on hot, humid days may be as great as five or six percent of body weight. Replacement of water without salt replacement may still result in dehydration, since one of the functions of salt is to hold water in suspension in the cells.

In laboratory studies, ingestion of up to a liter did not interfere with performance. For some athletes, the ingestion of larger amounts of water seemed to make them lazy, and the incentive or motive for good performance was then missing. Liquids other than water (isotonic liquids) have been marketed for their property of being assimilated more rapidly than water. Additional objective evidence of the advantages of this medium is still needed.

Altitude has an effect on physical performance

Anyone who read about, took part in, or watched the 1968 Olympics in Mexico City became aware of the effects of high altitude on performance. Whether the effects were physiological or psychological was at times hard to discern. One year in advance of the Olympics, seventy doctors from a number of participating countries were supposedly studying the effects of altitude in Mexico City.

Lung ventilation increases progressively with increases in altitude. The reduction in the partial pressure of oxygen necessitates breathing more air in the attempt to obtain the same amount of oxygen as at sea level. The amount of oxygen necessary for a given physical activity remains the same at all altitudes, but the increased work of the muscles of respiration requires the consumption of additional oxygen. At altitudes of about 7,000 feet, respiration may increase as much as one-third.

Without sufficient oxygen, heart rates for work increase and blood pressure rises. Short bursts of work are not affected if they are not dependent on oxygen uptake. This fact was well summarized by deVries:

> Not all athletic performances suffer because of the hypoxia of higher altitudes. Obviously "one maximal effort" activities such as shot put, long jump, high jump, etc., do not suffer because they do not depend upon O_2 transport. Furthermore, events of less than one minute duration, such as the 100 and 200 yard dashes, are also performed (very largely) anaerobically, and consequently they are unimpaired (but recovery times are longer).[1]

The human body has a remarkable ability to acclimatize to altitude as well as to heat. Although some individuals do not acclimatize readily, most begin to do so in about a week, and adjustment increases with additional time spent. This acclimatization lasts to some degree for a period of about one month after return to a lower altitude. Balke lists the factors in acclimatization to altitude changes.

> These mechanisms are: increased pulmonary ventilation with accompanying changes of the acid-base balance of the blood, improved diffusion capacity for oxygen in the lungs as manifested by a decrease

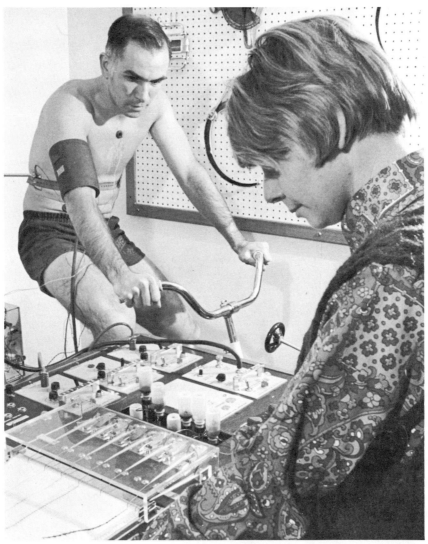

A six-channel physiograph during a physical work capacity test. Photo courtesy of Exercise Physiology Laboratory, Kent State University.

in the alveolar-arterial (A-a) gradient for oxygen, and the increase of the red blood cell count as well as the hemoglobin content of the blood.[2]

The physically fit individual has a greater aerobic capacity than the unfit individual

Aerobic work is a result of that process by which chemical energy is converted into muscular work with the utilization of oxygen and without the development of an oxygen debt. Several factors benefit physically

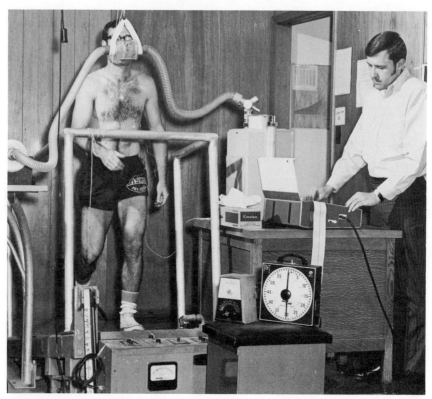

Measurement of oxygen uptake during treadmill running, with electrocardiograph monitoring. Photo courtesy of Exercise Physiology Laboratory, Kent State University.

fit individuals: (a) their hearts are larger because of their training; (b) their resting pulse rates are lower; (c) their stroke volumes (volume of blood expelled from the heart with each beat) are greater; (d) their capillary beds (number of capillaries per cubic centimeter of muscle tissue) are greater; and (e) the using muscle cell of the individual is able to utilize the available oxygen to a greater degree.

The reciprocal innervation of pairs of antagonistic muscles results in smooth and harmonious movement

According to deVries,

> In the case of the flexion reflex—in order that it might proceed with dispatch—the antagonistic extensor muscle group must be prevented from acting. This inhibition of the antagonists is accomplished by kinesthetic impulses from the muscle spindles of the flexor muscle and these synapse not only with the flexor motor neuron directly, but also, indirectly, with the motor neurons of extensor muscles of the same joint.[3]

Most athletic sports demand this type of smooth action. Hitting a golf ball or baseball, catching, shooting a basketball, and diving are examples. One needs only to go to an ice or roller skating arena to observe the defiance of this principle in action. The tightening of both sets of antagonistic muscles results in jerky and uncoordinated movement.

Outside stimuli, such as fear, pressure, cold, and criticism, can bring about undesirable results. For example, a beginner may hit a golf ball well, and yet, when faced with an obstacle such as a pond in front of the tee, may ignore the principle underlying the relaxing of antagonistic muscles.

Teaching and coaching which emphasize relaxation contribute to smoother performance of activities. Opportunities to play under less stressful situations and under game conditions can contribute to a relaxed performance.

At one time it was believed that heavy weight-lifting was detrimental to anyone who wished to perform in activities that demand smooth action. There has been no evidence to substantiate this belief.

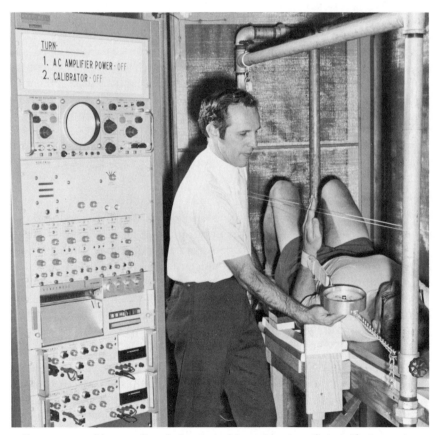

Electromyographic recording during test of isometric strength test. Photo courtesy of Electromyographic Laboratory, Kent State University.

Muscle tissue increases in size (hypertrophy) with increased use (work) and decreases in size (atrophy) with disuse
Normally called the overload principle of work, this principle is important in that there is a high correlation between increase in muscle size and increase in muscle strength, although there can in fact be an increase in strength without an increase in size. Increase in muscle size is due to an increase not in the number but in the size of fibers and the intramuscular tissue.

A muscle can be overloaded in either of two ways. When overloaded isotonically, the muscle shortens; when overloaded isometrically, the muscle remains the same in length. Advocates of both systems of exercise can be found. The muscles can be exercised isometrically by exertion, without equipment, against such immovable objects as walls and floors. The original investigators, Hettinger and Mueller, indicated that a maximum effect could be obtained by one six-second isometric contraction against two-thirds of an individual's maximum effort. Subsequent investigators have modified the number of seconds and the intensity of the effort. There are two important weaknesses of this system of muscle development: there is very little cardiovascular development, and the strength development may be restricted mainly to that one angle in the whole range of motion in a joint.

Isotonic exercise depends on the use of resistive exercise of submaximum effort with four to eight repetitions. The motivational factor is greater in isotonic exercises because the individual can see the changes more readily—that is, they can be more easily measured. A greater number of repetitions enhances the improvement of muscular endurance.

Physical conditioning brings about beneficial physiological changes
In addition to the changes already noted, vigorous physical exercise enhances the functioning of the body in a number of ways. Some are discussed in the following paragraphs.

1. The resting heart rate of a conditioned individual becomes slower and more efficient. This change occurs in the overall-conditioned athlete rather than in one conditioned to perform a single activity, such as lifting. The heart as an organ is probably efficient up to about 180 beats per minute. Conditioned individuals are able to perform many more difficult physical activities before their hearts reach that level than can those whose heart beats are 20 to 30 beats higher per minute while at rest. Although the average heart rate is approximately 76 to 78 beats per minute, the highly conditioned athlete may have a rate in the 40s.

2. The heart size of a conditioned individual increases with activity. Since the heart is made up of muscle tissue, the trained individual's heart, in addition to having better tonus, is expected to increase somewhat in size. Note, however, that this increase in size (hypertrophy) should not be confused with distension of the heart, which is pathological in nature.

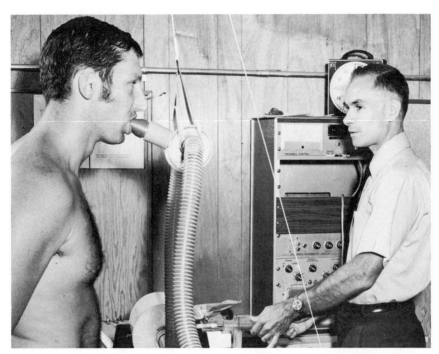

Measurement of cardiac output by the carbon dioxide rebreathing method. Photo courtesy of Exercise Physiology Laboratory, Kent State University.

3. The conditioned individual has a larger heart stroke volume than an unconditioned one. Stroke volume, the amount of blood ejected from the heart with each beat, increases slightly during exercise. A greater stroke volume, combined with an increase in heart size, results in the greater cardiac output necessary for the transportation of oxygen that will affect the delay of fatigue.

4. The conditioned athlete's total volume of blood and the amount of hemoglobin exceed those of the unconditioned individual. The volume may increase by as much as ten percent. Since the stroke volume partially depends on the blood volume available, this increase is beneficial in prevention and recovery from fatigue.

Common drugs may have an effect on physical performance

Since common drugs have varied physiological effects, we will examine them individually in terms of their benefits or deleterious effects. We will not deal here with illegal drugs, since their illegality should preclude their use.

1. Nicotine (as found in tobacco) has been the theme of many discussions and the basis of extensive research. The evidence that links smoking to lung cancer should be the overriding consideration in all of these

discussions. Although it is a stimulant, nicotine depresses the production of adrenalin and constricts the blood vessels (the smaller ones drastically). This factor has had a long-standing association with heart disease. A long period of smoking causes a pulmonary fibrosis (thickening of cells of the pulmonary tract). Smoking also causes an inhalation of carbon monoxide, which interferes with oxygen uptake. Although the effects of nicotine are temporary in nature, sufficient time should elapse to allow for its removal from the body before competition is attempted. There is no evidence whatsoever of benefits to justify its use.

2. Alcohol is a transitory stimulant and then becomes a depressant. It is also a vasodilator. Its first depressant effects are noticed in the judgment centers (frontal lobe) rather than in the motor centers of the brain. Stories of athletes who drank and still achieved greatness have been used as an argument for permissiveness with some athletes. The problem is complicated in certain communities, where ethnic groups use both wine and beer as part of their staple diet. Evidence does not warrant the use of a drug that can impair judgment.

3. Amphetamine sulfate is a stimulant to the nervous system. It raises the blood pressure and heart rate, and it retards the recovery of both. Golding and Barnard found that d-amphetamine sulfate had no significant effects on the performance of conditioned or unconditioned subjects in either the rested or the fatigued state.[4] Most other research has produced similar results. Evidence does not warrant use to enhance performance; such use may, in fact, interfere with the rest necessary to good performance.

4. Caffeine, an ingredient of both coffee and tea, is a vasoconstrictor and yet has a dilative effect on the coronary artery. It stimulates the central nervous system and does delay the onset of fatigue. There is some evidence that it may cause impairment in coordination (Graf), that larger than normal amounts of lactic acid appear from muscles exposed to caffeine, and that muscle metabolism (O_2 consumption) is elevated when it is present (Hartree and Hill.) As a diuretic, caffeine stimulates the kidneys and may increase production by several hundred percent. Since coffee and tea are consumed extensively in our culture, their use is almost impossible to control. Still, it need not be advocated.

5. Anabolic steroids are widely used by weight lifters, weight men in track, and football players. These commercial steroids have the same effect as does testosterone, which is produced in the normal male. There is some evidence that steroids have an effect on muscle strength and body weight when they are used in combination with an adequate protein diet and a program of weight training. The extent of these changes is now undergoing study. Unfortunately, there are several known and suspected side effects that raise serious doubts as to the wisdom of such use. Among them are the impairment of liver function, premature

cessation of long-bone growth in the prepubertal boy, change in size of testes, suppression of pituitary action, and acute muscular cramping during activity. Until more definite long-range findings are available, the use of anabolic steroids is hazardous at best.

There are a number of physiological and anatomical differences between the adult male and female which have a bearing on physical activity
The differences that may affect fatigue and recovery include the following.

1. The number of red blood cells (erythrocytes) per cubic millimeter is greater for males than for females. The male has approximately 5 million red blood cells, the female 4½ million.
2. The average male heart is larger than the average female heart.
3. The average heart rate of the male is lower than that of the female.
4. The average male has more hemoglobin per 100 millimeters of blood than does the average female.
5. The basal metabolic rate is higher for the male than for the female.
6. The cardiac cost of a work load is less for a male than for a female.
7. At a given work load, the oxygen uptake of the female is lower than that of the male.

The statements above reinforce the knowledge that the male has greater capacity to resist fatigue and recovers more rapidly from fatigue than the female.

SUMMARY

The purpose of presenting a selected number of anatomical and physiological principles is to provide knowledge about the body and its functions that is essential for a good teacher of physical education. Such knowledge sets the teacher apart from the technician, who may know how to do something without knowing the reasons for doing it. The knowledgeable physical educator can explain why exercise is good and how performance is enhanced when it is based on scientific principles. This background is the basis of good instruction.

STUDENT PROJECTS

1. Observe different athletic teams and record the positions filled by players with different body types.
2. If the department has a physiology and exercise laboratory, visit it and observe the types of activities under research.

GLOSSARY OF TERMS

Somatotyping Determination of body types by matching with a series of predetermined characteristics.

Aerobic Pertaining to work done by muscle with the utilization of oxygen.

Anaerobic Pertaining to work done by muscle without the utilization of oxygen and resulting in an oxygen debt.

Atrophy Reduction in muscle size due to lack of activity.

Hypertrophy Increase in muscle size due to activity.

Isotonic Pertaining to exercise that includes movement with resistance and a shortening of muscles.

Isometric Pertaining to exercise than includes resistance but no movement or change in muscle length.

REFERENCES

1. Herbert A. deVries, *Physiology of Exercise for Physical Education and Athletics.* (Dubuque, Iowa: Wm. C. Brown, 1974), pp. 328-329.
2. Harold B. Falls, ed., *Exercise Physiology* (New York: Academic Press, 1968), p. 249.
3. deVries, p. 34.
4. L. A. Golding and R. J. Barnard, "The Effect of d-Amphetamine Sulfate on Physical Performance," *Journal of Sports Medicine and Physical Fitness* **3** (December 1963), pp. 221–224

SELECTED READINGS

Astrand, Per-olof, and Rodahl, Kaare. *Textbook of Work Physiology.* New York: McGraw-Hill, 1970.

Basmajian, J. V. *Muscles Alive.* Baltimore: Williams and Wilkins, 1967.

Crouch, James E. *Functional Human Anatomy.* Philadelphia: Lea & Febiger, 1965.

deVries, Herbert A. *Physiology of Exercise for Physical Education and Athletics.* 2d ed. Dubuque, Iowa: Wm. C. Brown, 1974.

Edwards, Linder F. *Concise Anatomy.* New York: McGraw-Hill, 1956.

Falls, Harold B., ed. *Exercise Physiology.* New York: Academic Press, 1968.

Garden, John W.; Dodd, I. Wilson; and Rasch, P. J. "Acclimatization of Healthy Young Adult Males to a Hot-Wet Environment." *Journal of Applied Physiology* **21** (March 1966), pp. 665–669.

Gaslen, R. V.; Balke, B.; Nagle, F. J.; and Phillips, E. E. "Effects of Some Tranquilizing Analeptic and Vasodilating Drugs on Physical Work Capacity and Orthostatic Tolerance." *Aerospace Medicine* **35** (July 19, 1964), pp. 630–633.

Golding, L. A., and Barnard, R. J. "The Effects of d-Amphetamine Sulfate on Physical Performance." *Journal of Sports Medicine and Physical Fitness* **3** (December 1963), pp. 221–224.

Karpovich, Peter V., and Sinning, Wayne. *Physiology of Muscular Activity*. 7th ed. Philadelphia: W. B. Saunders, 1971.

Lapp, Milton C., and Gee, Gink. "Human Acclimatization to Cold Water Immersion—Effects on Physiological Activities." *Archives of Environmental Health* **15** (November 1967), pp. 568–579.

Leary, W. P., and Wyndham, C. H. "Possible Effect on Athletic Performance of Mexico City's Altitude." *South African Medical Journal* **40** (November 1966), pp. 984–985.

Matthews, Donald K., and Fox, Edward L. *The Physiological Basis of Physical Education and Athletics*. Philadelphia: W. B. Saunders, 1971.

Reeves, John T.; Jokl, Peter; and Coln, Jerome. "Performance of Olympic Runners at Altitudes of 7,350 and 5,350 Feet." *The American Review of Respiratory Diseases* **92** (November 1965), pp. 813–816.

Stern, M. H., and Melville, K. I. "A Comparative Evaluation of the Action of Depressant and Stimulant Drugs on Human Performance." *Psychopharmacologia* **6** (1964), pp. 173–177.

Veghte, G. H., and Webb, Paul. "Body Cooling and Response to Heat." *Journal of Applied Physiology* **16** (March 1969), pp. 235–238.

Chapter 6
Foundations in the Behavioral Sciences

The behavioral sciences are one of the major intellectual and cultural inventions

BERNARD BERELSON

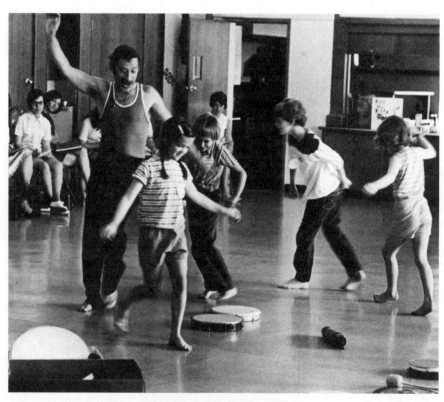

Skill acquisition is a function of early learning experiences.

JUST as it is necessary for prospective physical educators to familiarize themselves with the various biochemical, anatomical, and physiological principles so important to the discipline encompassing human movement, so it is necessary for them to become aware of the sociological and psychological principles which together constitute a part of the behavioral sciences.

The fields collectively embraced in what are termed the *behavioral sciences* represent a relatively new area of specialization, aimed primarily at understanding human behavior. Each individual behaves as an individual; nevertheless, given certain sets of circumstances, behavioral scientists make predictions of behavior patterns, with varying degrees of accuracy. Further, theories have been developed which explain certain human behavioral patterns with great accuracy. Regardless of the complexities surrounding it, human behavior can be researched scientifically.

The implications of the behavioral sciences for physical education are many and quite obvious. Sports situations often foster distinctive types of social behavior, and research that is being conducted increasingly in sports psychology and sports sociology helps to provide insight into such behavior. Why does a varsity team with all the physical requirements and skill to play well and win suffer through a disastrous season? Conversely, why does a participant who lacks what seem to be necessary physical attributes achieve success in a competitive situation in which he or she has no apparent chance? Why are teachers confronted with different degrees of success in two different but supposedly homogeneous groups when they use the same methodology with both? The answers to these questions fall within the purview of the behavioral sciences.

Since the behavioral sciences are of relatively recent origin, it is well to describe briefly their formulation and present status as well as to note their potential to physical education as a field of specialization. The broad term *social sciences* comprises three of the branches of learning which together make up the behavioral sciences: psychology, sociology, and anthropology. Berelson contends that any precise delineation of what constitutes the behavioral sciences is impossible. However, he states that two basic criteria must be met if a field is to be considered a part of the behavioral sciences: it must deal with human behavior, and it must conduct its study in a scientific manner to produce empirical, verifiable evidence.[1]

Examples of research in psychology which satisfy the above criteria include formulation of learning theory, exploration of personality, and experiments in communication. In sociology, the subject matter studied has included race relations and differing value orientations within a community. Analyses of cultural influences within and among ethnic groups are typical problems researched in anthropology. There are obvious overlaps among the three areas, but they are probably desirable rather than otherwise, since they indicate common concern about mutual problems, not mere proliferation.

Examples of research problems in physical education by specialists in the three social sciences are the relationships between social class and activity preference, the effect of audience on individual performance, and the function of sports in various primitive and modern societies.

Although the *discipline* of behavioral science is structurally very young, the vast number of topics germane to it and the resulting expansion of knowledge have given rise to another area of specialized study—social psychology—which is of great interest to physical education and from which we can broaden our discipline's horizons. *Social psychology* is the study of individuals and their behavioral dependence and interdependence in social and cultural settings. As the name implies, specialists in this area delimit their concerns neither psychologically nor sociologically; instead they recognize that human personality and behavior are results of both psychological processes and social influences. Social psychologists do not universally agree on a methodology for studying human social nature, but they are unanimous in their conviction that they can, through careful study, reveal our social nature and that such revelation will aid in understanding the human being in relation to the complex social forces that come into play.[2]

How does the discipline of physical education relate to the discipline of social psychology? It is indeed interesting to note that the first experimental observation in social psychology, made in 1898 by Triplett, not only dealt with the effects of competition on human performance, but also involved recreational skills, namely, riding bicycles and winding fishing reels. Triplett's general finding was that competition facilitated performance, that individuals performed better in competition than alone. What he then called "competition," however, is today known as "social facilitation."[3] Three concerns that are important to the social psychologist are also very important to the physical educator: competition, cooperation, and conflict. Surely an insight into the characteristics of one or all of these behavior traits would be beneficial to specialists in both areas. The physical educator who is most concerned with human behavior in a sociocultural context may well pursue a specialization in social psychology in his or her graduate work.

Knowledge today is so complex and so intricate that "strict disciplinarians" could never research innumerable ramifications of their discipline within narrow confines; they would not wish to even if they could. The time is past when thoughtful academicians jealously guarded their discipline against what they considered encroachment by less well-prepared "outsiders." Reasonable people today realize that it is educationally desirable for different but related disciplines to conduct interdisciplinary investigations. Therefore, we find specialists within the discipline of physical education who, though primarily interested in physical education, have secondary interests that lie naturally within another and sometimes entirely different discipline. As an example, perhaps the relationship between the behavioral sciences and physical education is not so readily apparent as the relationship between medicine and physical education.

It is impossible in a book of this nature to explore fully the relationship between the behavioral sciences and physical education, but it is not impossible to help the beginning professional student in physical education become familiar with some of the more obvious connections between the two disciplines. Consequently, the remainder of this chapter will be devoted to a discussion of the history and current status of sports psychology and sports sociology and selected principles from psychology and sociology, together with their application to physical education. No principles will be listed as social-psychological since such a category would cut across both fields, and the precise delineation they would require is beyond the scope of this book.

PSYCHOLOGY, SPORT PSYCHOLOGY, AND PSYCHOLOGICAL PRINCIPLES

Although the beginnings of psychology can perhaps be traced back to Pluto and Aristotle and their discussions of mind-body relationships, experimental psychology as such is less than a century old. Many of the first problems scientifically researched revolved around theories of learning, motor learning, psychological conditioning, motivation, motor responses, and perception, all of which are also significant in physical education.

Although sport psychology per se can be traced back to the genesis of psychology as a discipline, much of the impetus in this area, particularly in the United States, has come about since World War II.[4] Sport psychologists today research such things as motivation, including the phenomenon of "psyching up" athletes (team arousal), and the role of personality in sports. Motivation to achieve success, for example, is not always predicated on a desire for the rewards which accrue to the winner; the motivation to avoid failure and its consequent unpleasantness is just as strong in some persons.[5]

As for the subject of arousing the emotions of a team, some sport psychologists today state that the relationship between arousal and performance is so complex that the coach is best advised not to experiment with techniques that may prove, if not actually harmful, at least not beneficial. Griffith, the "father of sport psychology," believed that emotional arousal did not affect performance positively, and he recorded that Knute Rockne, the fabled Notre Dame coach, agreed with this theory.[6] Ostensibly, however, this view is not shared by many of the foreign coaches and psychologists. Vanek and Cratty believe that "future records will be broken primarily because of increased attention to the psychological parameters of human personality."[7] It seems nonetheless apparent not only that different tasks demand different levels of arousal for the best performance, but that different personalities respond differently (sometimes adversely) to arousal. Since it is difficult to determine accurately the arousal level of an individual or a team at any given time, the need for research in these areas seems acute.[8] Future sport psychologists, take note! The potential contribution of such research to sports and organized athletics is monumental.[9]

Personality and its relationship to ability in sports is another area in which a high degree of research sophistication is needed. Physical educators and coaches, who have long expounded on the desirable personality traits exhibited by athletes, tend to imply that such traits are a result of participation in sports. Perhaps, however, these remarkable personality traits were present *before* participation. Again, future sport psychologists, take note!

It is probably correct to say that initial consideration of psychological theory by physical educators was along the lines of learning theories, principles, and "laws," as advocated by educational psychologists. This application was only natural in that the long-term concern of physical education was to prove that the two words which entitle our discipline are neither mutually exclusive nor contradictory.

Psychological Principles

A selected few of the psychological principles related to learning are described below, and an attempt is made to relate the application of each principle to physical education.

Individuals do not all learn at the same rate or in the same manner

If this principle were not true, the teaching of any subject would be remarkably simple. Any brilliant educational psychologist could develop a teaching model with clearly defined directions, which any reasonably intelligent *technician* could follow with guaranteed results. However, the principle is true, and we therefore need to explore its many ramifications.

The key word is "individuals." Since every learner is an individual, he or she is cast from a unique mold. His or her personality, environment, innate intellectual as well as motor capacity—these are but examples of what makes one different from all others. Knowing that every person is unique but also that every learner experiences "plateaus" (leveling off in the learning curve where no further learning occurs) and "dips" (regressions) in learning, the wise teacher realizes the need for motivating the student so that the dips in the learning rate can be avoided and the length of the plateaus decreased. In physical education, teachers may try rivalry as a motivating device, although they should be cognizant of the fact that the effectiveness of this technique decreases with the age of the learner. With a group of high school age, teachers may try praise as a positive reinforcement to learning. For certain motor tasks, however, reproof has been demonstrated to facilitate learning more than praise. Although the literature from reinforcement studies tends to demonstrate that a combination of positive and negative reinforcement techniques (with a heavy emphasis on positive) is most productive, not even the psychologist can predict which forms of motivation will work when and under what set of circumstances. Teaching, therefore, is not "remarkably simple"!

The learner repeats reactions which are satisfying and avoids those which are not

This is the old "law of effect," which today might be more appropriately discussed under a "reinforcement" theory. Indeed, the statement is so true that it hardly requires explanation; but, as often happens, it may be overlooked simply because it is obvious.

For example, some football coaches, usually neophytes in the coaching ranks, are so imbued with a "let's-separate-the-men-from-the-boys" attitude that they conduct vigorous physical scrimmages almost from the beginning of the football season. The coach who does so fails to realize that there are undoubtedly some boys, at least among his beginners, who are not yet certain whether they like physical contact. To expose them to such contact too soon may make some of them decide not to continue in football. A more reasonable coach brings his boys along slowly and tries to make each practice session satisfying. Thereby he more nearly ensures that potentially good players will remain with football long enough to achieve their potential. A more dramatic example of the working of this principle is the beginning swimmer who "almost drowns." Once such an unpleasant experience has occurred, it is difficult for the learner to reenter the water and enjoy learning to swim.

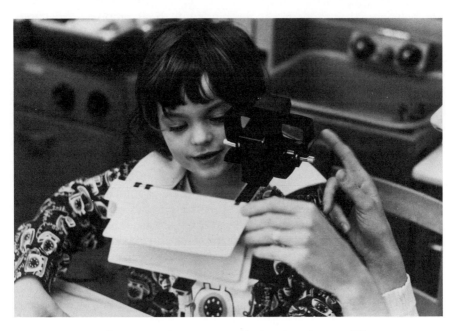

Visual perception is important in the learning of motor skill.

A reaction will not transfer to all situations

Again, if this statement were not true, teaching would be considerably easier. An insightful learner *may* see the relationship between skill in different activities, and insight is positively correlated with intelligence. Regardless of the intelligence level of the individual, however, he or she can profit from teacher guidance in the matter of transfer.

In physical education there seems to be a direct relationship between the skill components of, say, an overhand softball throw and a tennis serve. Why, then, should not the teacher cite this relationship to the individual having difficulty with the tennis serve? There is a strong chance that this same learner has long since learned the overhand throw. The application of this principle seems to be that if the teacher wants transfer to occur, he or she should teach it. Such teaching can take two forms. In the first and most desirable form, an individual can be taught in such a way that cognitive outcomes are ensured from the beginning of the organized physical education instruction. Thus, the student *understands* the mechanical principles underlying efficient movement and is able to apply them to any new situation. Sometimes, however, even individuals who have been taught this way have trouble with a new skill for any one of a number of reasons. Therefore, the teacher may on occasion have to resort to the second form of teaching and point out the similarities between the two skills. Direct teaching, or what Mosston refers to as "command" teaching, cannot always be avoided.[10]

Habit represents an important factor in learning

All learning theories deal in one way or another with habit, whether they are behavioristic-connectionist theories, with their emphasis on conditioning, or cognitive-field theories, with their emphasis on conceptual processes. One can assume that the various behavioristic theories place greater stress on habit formation, but in any case, repetition of a motor task is essential if performance of the task is to become automatic. Nevertheless, current research in motor learning indicates that two basic types of motor skills must be differentiated: *open,* where the environment is variable and changing and the response is *to* the environment; and *closed,* where the environment is stable and the response is *on* the environment.

In physical education, automatic or habitual motor responses are no doubt desirable at the lower level of skill development as well as for closed skills. This circumstance explains the emphasis on drill that characterizes much of the teaching seen in the gymnasium or on the playing fields. For more complex, open motor tasks, however, dependence on habitual response alone is sheer folly. If automatic performance of a complex, open task depends on the existence of a certain combination of external conditions, the wise teacher recognizes the necessity for stressing cognitive concepts and alternative responses, because that particular combination of conditions of the external environment may only seldom occur.

In basketball, for example, we often find players who have not only favorite shots but favorite spots on the floor from which to shoot. The coach who is cognizant of motor learning theory, whether or not he or she is working with a patterned offense, not only teaches the squad variations of "plays" but even goes so far as to have the guards double-team the player who always wants to get to that favorite spot before shooting. Since the coach recognizes that the opposing coach may be teaching exactly the same strategy, he or she tries to prepare the player for the fact that one's pet shot from a pet spot will not always work. In other words, the coach tries to get the players to understand and conceptualize the different situations as they occur on the floor and to adjust to them accordingly. However, the free-throw, a closed-type skill, demands habitual, consistent response for proficiency. It can be seen, then, that a consideration of open or closed type skills demands different learning and practice procedures.

Psychological tensions are produced by certain situations

There is some degree of tension in any learning situation, but some individuals reach much more quickly than others the level of psychological tension that minimizes learning or even precludes it. Such factors as noise, physical condition, temperature of the room, emotional status, personality, and presence of others contribute to tension in varying degrees.

The wise teacher should be aware of rising psychological tension, whether in one individual, a few, or the entire class. He or she also needs to know what to do about it, but unfortunately, there is no universal solution. From experience the teacher learns to know each individual better and thus becomes more able to cope with the situation. For example, he or she may talk to an individual away from the group, completely change the learning activity, or strive to adjust physical factors to improve the environment.

Learning is a process experiencing and responding to a variety of situations

This principle is of great importance in all cognitive-field theories of learning, but it is valid in the behavioristic theories as well. No learning situation can be so isolated that other situations do not enter the total picture. Even those theoreticians who believe in the part method of teaching still admit that the learning of isolated competent parts does not always produce an effective performance in the whole (game) situation. It therefore seems wise for the physical educator to teach in game-like situations.

"Gamelike" does not mean throwing the ball out and just letting the learners play, however, It implies a concerted effort on the part of the teacher to help the learner conceptualize the relationship between the "parts" and the "whole." It further means that, on occasion, practice of a skill is conducted under conditions that duplicate as closely as possible the actual game situation. For example, to keep practicing the bully in

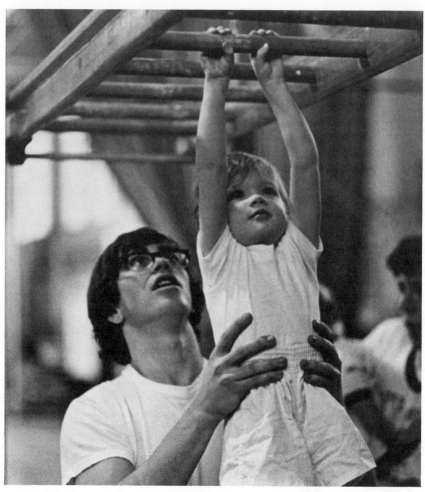

Manual guidance can be an appropriate technique in the learning of motor skills.

field hockey with only the two center forwards involved is rather futile when, in a game situation, the "bullyer" is immediately confronted by several other girls.

Feedback is essential for effective learning of motor skills

There are two types of feedback (information sources) which are extremely important when attempting to learn a motor skill: knowledge of performance, which relates to movement qualities, and knowledge of results (KR), which relates to goal attainment of the movement. Both of these can be conveyed through internal (individual or task) or external (external to the task; in practice, predominantly the teacher) sources. External sources are more important at the beginning of skill learning, whereas internal sources seem to be more important at the later stages of learning.

Exactly what method should be used to relay feedback to the learner cannot be defined explicitly because of the complexity of the variables involved, although in general more specific feedback results in greater learning. The physical education teacher should be ever cognizant of the necessity to furnish the student with feedback as quickly and as specifically as possible, along with an understanding of its *cause*. In other words, students should be taught from the beginning of their organized physical education experience to understand the principles of movement so that, given knowledge of results, they can correct errors and improve their performance.

The psychological principles presented here are only a few of the many principles that are germane to the work of the teacher-coach. As students of physical education delve more deeply into their professional studies, they should gain greater knowledge of psychology and thus greater insight into the psychological principles on which teaching is based. As Scott so well states, the physical educator is a "practical psychologist" who contributes to the following psychological outcomes as well as to skill acquisition: changed attitudes, improved social efficiency, improved mental health, improved sensory perception and responses, and improved ability to relax.[11]

SOCIOLOGY, SPORT SOCIOLOGY, AND SOCIOLOGICAL PRINCIPLES

A significant book edited by Loy and Kenyon constitutes the first attempt to bring together in English a representative sampling of the wide variety of studies relating to both sociology and physical education that are being conducted throughout the world.[12] A more recent effort by Ball and Loy continues in that vein and treats particular topics within the sociology of sport in greater depth.[13] Both books are perhaps basic to anyone desiring further information in the area.

Sociology can be defined as the "scientific study of society, its structure, functions, and processes."[14] It can be divided into three broad fields: study of groups, analysis of institutions, and study of general social structure. Although the "discipline" was founded in the nineteenth century, those features which make sociology truly a discipline—rigorous scientific methodology, behavioral orientation, conceptual consciousness—are to a great extent the product of the past fifty years.[15]

Currently sociologists are very active in researching various problems that come under the general classification of group study, such as types of social groups, patterns of relationships between and among groups, bases on which groups are formulated, and attitudes within groups. Sociological research in the field of institutional analysis has fostered the formulation of ideas concerning, for example, the persistence of such basic institutions as the family, the interdependence of institutions as seen from the fact that change in one presages changes in others, and the tendency of groups to perpetuate themselves. Social structure in general can best be understood by a careful appraisal of the social classes within the overall structure. Along these lines, sociologists have been researching such factors as expected behavior characteristics within classes, stresses that arise between classes, and mobility between and within classes.[16]

One can easily see how the concerns above are related to a study of sports, play, and games, and thus one can readily understand that a subdiscipline known as sport sociology soon established itself in the academic community.

Some of the early leaders in the field of physical education in the United States mentioned in Chapter 1, such as Hetherington and Williams, asserted social objectives for physical education as early as the turn of this century. Nevertheless, there were few attempts by social scientists to study sports, which make up one of our most common yet least understood social institutions. Most of the scientific study in this area has been conducted within the past 20 to 25 years. The efforts have not been confined to the United States; in fact, serious study of play, sports, and games in foreign countries preceded similar activity here.

Sociological literature pertaining to sports is not confined to sociologists or physical educators. Indeed, a recent article by Bill Russell, the basketball great, has sociological, psychological, and philosophical overtones.[17] And, of course, journalistic literature abounds in discussions of the relationships of sports to society.

In 1959 the International Council of Sport and Physical Education was formed, and in 1964 that UNESCO-sponsored body appointed a Committee on Sport Sociology. The committee comprises both physical educators and sociologists, and the programs its members support have exhibited a diversified international flavor and continue to do so. The committee has sponsored international seminars, and it coordinates international research on the subject as well as publishes *The International Review of Sport Sociology.*

The number of persons in the United States who might properly be called sport sociologists is small; however, there is encouraging evidence that interest in this subdiscipline is growing in the fact that the number of institutions of higher learning that offer specialized study in the area, both at the master's and the doctoral level, is increasing. That the field of sociology per se is accepting the sport sociologist as a well-prepared disciplinarian is in turn demonstrated by the fact that there is also an increase in the number of courses cross-listed in departments of physical education and sociology that are being taught by physical educators.

Of the almost limitless possibilities for research in the area, just a few are cited below.

1. *The role of sports and games in influencing value systems and the converse.* For example, has the "All-American" hero type vanished with the emergence professional athletes who see their role strictly in business terms?

2. *Influences of sports on family life.* Many people believe that the family that prays together stays together. Many physical educators would like to believe as well that the family that *plays* together stays together. Is this true?

3. *Social phenomena surrounding sports events.* How do social phenomena differ with different events? For example, contrast a boxing match with, say, a "tailgate" picnic prior to an Ivy League football game.

4. *The role of politics and government in athletic endeavors.* Should governments subsidize Olympic competitors? Should the International Olympic Committee ban any nation from competing because of its internal political structure?

5. *The role of sports in developing countries.* Why does the Peace Corps recruit so heavily among physical educators and athletes?

6. *Crowd behavior.* Why is an unruly mob "tolerated" after a big football victory, when the same mob actions in different situations would earn for the participating college-age youths the label of "radicals"?

7. *Values in sports that serve as instruments for the social good.* Has the rise of organized sports in the United States lessened intolerance and discrimination?

Sociological Principles

As before, when dealing with the psychological aspects of the behavioral sciences spectrum, we now offer a selected few sociological principles together with their application to physical education. Though limited, the list is fairly representative.

The social situation inflences the learning process
The child in a learning situation is confronted by many social factors, some of them contradictory. In the matter of value orientation alone, for example, an educator or family member who espouses the value of honesty may on occasion be observed in dishonest behavior. What is the child to conclude in regard to his or her own actions?

The physical educator must not only teach those social values deemed desirable in our culture, but practice them under all circumstances.

Peer-group attitudes are important behavior-forming influences
That this statement is more true at certain maturation stages than at others is uncontestable. Peer-group influence is usually at its height at the junior high school level, when the importance to all youngsters of being accepted by their peers tends to be so great that they will conform to expected behavior patterns, even if they question them, in order to maintain status in the group. This phenomenon explains such diverse things as

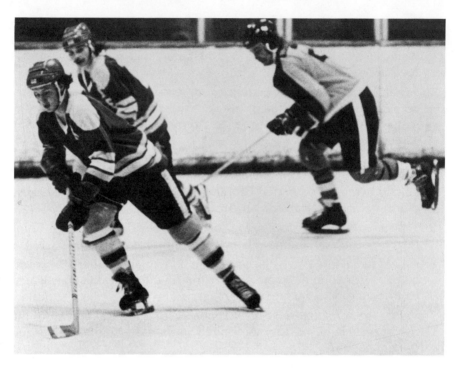

Appropriate expression of aggressive behavior may be learned through participation in physical education and sport.

fads in clothing and hair styles or the conforming to certain moral standards, even though they are contrary to deep-seated religious convictions.

The role the leaders of the peer group play can be crucial. If they have values that society defines as desirable, no problem exists. If they have values that point in the opposite direction, however, it is the duty of the physical educator to try to change their value system, thereby influencing the entire group. For example, a leader who feels that a certain activity is too "square" can influence the group to resist. Unfortunately, many athletic coaches today are faced with the job of "selling" interscholastic participation.

Each person should have an opportunity for self-realization within bounds that society deems desirable

Self-realization has always been an objective in American education—an objective that often receives only lip service. Today, with the behavioral sciences stressing the importance of self-realization, many people believe that society is going overboard in not only allowing but encouraging everyone "to do your own thing." Experience in similar circumstances suggests that vacillating from one end of the conformity-permissiveness continuum to the other is unproductive. Such a procedure, in fact, often leads not only to a more perplexed and perhaps less stable individual, but also to a society seemingly without direction.

The implication for physical educators, then, is clear although their task is nonetheless difficult. They must provide the individual with an opportunity for genuine self-realization. Perhaps they can best do this by offering a wide variety of activities in the program so that each individual can find at least one in which he or she can excel. Lessening the stress on the authoritarian teaching which has characterized our field should also prove beneficial in the implementation of self-realization.

Education should stress the concept of sharing

The United States is a nation of contrast, not the least of which is great wealth and abject poverty. If American society values the concept of sharing, education must do more than merely provide lip service about it. The various fields in education must provide opportunities for sharing and must stress the value cognitively so that the transfer of sharing from one situation to another is enhanced.

Physical education, with its emphasis on the concept of teamwork, is a particularly good field in which to meet this objective. But if sharing is to become truly a behavorial outcome and not merely a paper objective, physical educators need to point out how teamwork can logically transfer to other life situations, in spite of the fact that transfer is usually situation-specific. There are many instances in sports in which victory depends on subordinating oneself for the good of the group—sacrificing in baseball, passing off to a teammate in basketball, setting up for a spike in volleyball. In these instances, race, color, creed, and economic status, to cite just a few factors, are immaterial. Why shouldn't they be immaterial in life?

Education should help each individual adjust successfully to changing social conditions

Perhaps the need for such help has never been more obvious than in today's society. Not only is there a "generation gap," but there seems also to be sincere confusion about standards and values among school-age individuals in an existentially oriented environment. Education must rise to the challenge and become an effective tool for resolving conflicts.

If physical education is to fit into this changed social order, the curriculum must escape the traditional, repetitive, practical approach and develop an orientation toward more diversified exploration of human movement. Perhaps the current emphasis on movement education and problem-solving methodology is a step in this direction. Along with a change in the program of activities must come a change in the philosophy regarding the learner's role in the educative process. Youth needs to be taught how to cope intelligently with differing viewpoints, differing abilities, differing life-styles. What better place to do this than the laboratory-activity sessions that characterize much of the learning process in physical education, where there is truly an intermingling of many and diverse personalities and viewpoints? In contrast to the too-typical classroom situation where social problems are merely verbalized, the physical education laboratory affords an opportunity to put theory into practice.

The principles we have cited here, though few in number, are representative of those sociological precepts which physical educators should use to guide their actions when dealing with possible social learning. These selected principles should assume additional importance as the prospective teachers' exposure to the study of sociology becomes broader and more diversified.

SUMMARY

Physical educators have long insisted that desirable social and psychological traits are natural outcomes from work in the discipline. Although such claims seem to have merit, research into cause-and-effect relationships is greatly needed to establish the validity of assumptions about the behavioral consequences of participation in physical education and sports.

Research into the psychology of physical education and sports is needed to provide insight into such diverse psychological manifestations as motivation; emotional arousal and its effects on performance; self-actualization and all its contiguous aspects, such as ego fulfillment, self-perception, etc.; the role of play in mental health; theories of play; the attraction of spectator sports; cooperation versus competition; eu-stress versus dys-stress;[18] and personality.

Personality factors have interested physical educators for many years and continue to be the subject of psychological research in physical education. Such research has in the past left much to be desired in terms of rigorous scientific methodology, and therefore the conclusions have been, at best, generalized and superficial.[19] There is hope that this situation is changing, because physical educators with specialized training in psychology are beginning to realize that there is a vast, untapped well of insight into the complexities of personality and physical activity waiting to be revealed by sophisticated research. Many universities today are offering courses in motor learning and the psychology of sports. Furthermore, the founding in 1965 of the North American Society of Psychology in Sport and Physical Activity, which sponsors national and international congresses of sports psychology,[20] and the publication of such journals as the *International Journal of Sport Psychology*, the *Journal of Motor Behavior*, and the *Psychology of Sport and Motor Behavior* are indications that this speciality within the discipline of physical education has established itself.

Snyder, a sociologist engaged in research on aspects of the sociology of sports, states that the dimensions of social interaction in the socialization process must be analyzed in order to understand whether the influence of participation in physical education and sports activities can be diffused beyond a specific situation.[21] The following dimensions in the specific situational context are among the most important, according to Snyder.

1. *The participants' degree of involvement in the activity.* There is usually greater involvement in a varsity sport than in a physical education class. The coach and captain of a particular varsity team also tend to be more deeply involved than substitute players are.

2. *Voluntary or involuntary selection of and participation in an activity.* Participation in varsity sports is usually voluntary, whereas participation in the physical education program is required. One would expect the voluntary activity to foster greater involvement and thus a more diffused socialization.

3. *Instrumental or socialization relationships.* This dimension relates to the quality of the relationship between participants and socializing agents. Instrumental relationships can be thought of as largely utiltarian with no intervening variables. In contrast, socialization relationships foster genuine interplay among participants and are thus personally satisfying ends in themselves. Socialization relationships are difficult, if not impossible, to encourage in a traditionally taught class in physical education. The teacher who is concerned with developing this type of relationship needs to be cognizant of the shortcomings of the "traditional" method of teaching.

4. *The power and prestige of the teacher or coach.* It seems obvious that the higher the esteem in which the teacher is held, the greater his or her influence will be. Power is akin to esteem or prestige, and generally speaking, the person who is held in high esteem also exerts great control over the participants.

5. *Social and personal characteristics of the participants.* Such traits as physical talent, mental ability, and self-perception are important in the diffusion of behavioral outcomes; nevertheless, such variables as social class and ethnic affiliations must not be overlooked.

Snyder concludes by asserting that physical educators must understand the socialization process that occurs in physical education and that attention to this consideration must receive high priority within the discipline.

Just as psychology and sociology of physical education and sports have emerged as recognized subdisciplines of their parent disciplines, so social psychology as an interdisciplinary field has become of extreme importance in the body of knowledge germane to the discipline of physical education. Martens contends that social psychology is primarily concerned with the process of social influence and that as an area of study it is distinct from either psychology or sociology in that it is primarily interested in understanding the social-influence processes underlying the *individual* as a participant in social relationships.[22]

In conclusion, the social sciences which together constitute the behavioral sciences abound in research possibilities in physical education and sports. But only when physical educators use the particular research designs and techniques rigorously and well will we be able to do more than conjecture about the interrelationships among those disciplines interested in people and their activities.

STUDENT PROJECTS

1. Interview various coaches at both the high school and college level to determine whether they believe in "psyching up" their teams. If they do, what methods do they use? If they do not believe in it, why not?
2. Repeat the above with several varsity players.
3. Report on at least one *research* study on the general topic of personality of the athlete.
4. What sports in the United States seem to have ethnic connotations? Why?
5. Select some good bowlers and some nonbowlers from the class. Have both groups bowl one string without an audience and record their scores. Repeat with the entire class as an audience. Observe the results and try to explain them.
6. Divide the class into two groups. Have the members of the first group throw beanbags ten feet over their shoulders into a waste basket. Record the number of successes in a ten-second time span. Immediately repeat the test twice. Now have the second group perform the same test, but give them a five-minute break between test trials. Observe the results and try to explain them.

GLOSSARY OF TERMS

Behavioral sciences   Those fields which attempt to understand human behavior, including psychology, sociology, and anthropology.

Social psychology   The study of individuals and their behavioral dependence and independence in social and cultural settings.

Sport psychology   The study of the influences that produce regularities and diversities of human behavior in physical activity and sports settings.

Sport sociology   The study of sports as a social and cultural phenomenon.

Competition   A striving by two or more individuals or teams for one goal. As one individual or team moves toward that goal, the possibility that the others will reach it decreases.

Contest   A striving by two or more units (individuals or teams) for superiority under well-defined rules and mutual agreement.

Team arousal   An attempt to motivate a team to perform well, often called "psyching up."

REFERENCES

1. Bernard Berelson, ed., *The Behavioral Sciences Today* (New York: Harper & Row, 1964), p. 2.

2. William W. Lambert and Wallace E. Lambert, *Social Psychology* (Englewood Cliffs, N.J.: Prentice-Hall, 1964), pp. 4–6.

3. Norman Triplett, "The Dynamogenic Factors of Pacemaking and Competition," *American Journal of Psychology* **9** (1898), pp. 507–533.

4. Miroslav Vanek and Bryant J. Cratty, *Psychology and the Superior Athlete* (New York: Macmillan, 1970), pp. 3–32.

5. Don R. Bethe and Joe D. Willis, "Achievement Motivation: Implications for Physical Activity," *Quest* **13** (January 1970), pp. 18–22.

6. Walter Kroll and Guy Lewis, "America's First Sport Psychologist," *Quest* **13** (January 1970), p. 2.

7. Vanek and Cratty, p. 4.

8. Joseph B. Oxendine, "Emotional Arousal and Motor Performance," *Quest* **13** (January 1970), pp 23–32.

9. Bryant J. Cratty, "Coaching Decisions and Research in Sport Psychology," *Quest* **13** (January 1970), pp. 46–53.

10. Muska Mosston, *Teaching Physical Education: From Command to Discovery* (Columbus, Ohio: Charles E. Merrill, 1966).

11. M. Gladys Scott, "The Contributions of Physical Activity to Psychological Development," in *Anthology of Contemporary Readings,* eds. H. S. Slusher and A. S. Lockhart (Dubuque, Iowa: W. C. Brown, 1970), p. 130.

12. John W. Loy, Jr., and Gerald S. Kenyon, eds., *Sport, Culture, and Society* (New York: Macmillan, 1969).

13. Donald W. Ball and John W. Loy, *Sport and Social Order: Contributions to the Sociology of Sport* (Reading, Mass.: Addison-Wesley, 1975.)

14. Harry S. Alpert, "Sociology: Its Present Interests," in *The Behavioral Sciences Today,* ed. B. Berelson (New York: Harper & Row, 1964), p. 53

15. Ibid., p. 52.

16. Ibid., pp. 54–57.

17. William F. Russell, "Success Is a Journey," *Sports Illustrated* **32**:23 (June 8, 1970), pp. 80–88, 93.

18. Dorothy V. Harris, "On the Brink of Catastrophe," *Quest* **13** (January 1970), pp. 33–40.

19. Pearl Berlin, "Prolegomena to the Study of Personality by Physical Educators," *Quest* **13** (January 1970), pp. 54–63.

20. Vanek and Cratty, pp. 23–24.

21. Eldon E. Snyder, "Aspects of Socialization in Sports and Physical Education," *Quest* **14** (June 1970), pp. 1–7.

22. Rainer Martens, "A Social Psychology of Physical Activity," *Quest* **14** (June 1970), pp. 8–17.

SELECTED READINGS

Alpert, Harry S. "Sociology: Its Present Interests." In *The Behavioral Sciences Today*, edited by B. Berelson. New York: Harper & Row, 1964

Ball, Donald W., and Loy, John W. *Sport and Social Order: Contributions to Sociology of Sport*. Reading, Mass.: Addison-Wesley, 1975.

Bell, Virginia Lee. *Sensorimotor Learning*. Pacific Palisades: Goodyear, 1970.

Berelson, Bernard, ed. *The Behavioral Sciences Today*. New York: Harper & Row, 1964.

Berlin, Pearl. "Prolegomena to the Study of Personality by Physical Educators." *Quest* **13** (January 1970).

Bethe, Don R., and Willis, Joe D. "Achievement Motivation: Implications for Physical Activity." *Quest* **13** (January 1970).

Committee of Sport Sociology of the International Council of Sport and Physical Education, ed. *International Review of Sport Sociology*, Vols. 1, 2, 3. Warsaw: Polish Scientific, 1966, 1967, 1968.

Cratty, Bryant J. "Coaching Decisions and Research in Sport Psychology." *Quest* **13** (January 1970), pp. 46–53.

Drowatsky, John N. *Motor Learning Principles and Practices*. Minneapolis: Burgess, 1975.

Frost, Reuben B. *Psychological Concepts Applied to Physical Education and Coaching*. Reading, Mass.: Addison-Wesley, 1971.

Harris, Dorothy V. "On the Brink of Catastrophe." *Quest* **13** (January 1970).

Kroll, Walter, and Lewis, Guy M. "America's First Sport Psychologist." *Quest* **13** (January 1970).

Lambert, William W., and Lambert, Wallace E. *Social Psychology*. Englewood Cliffs, N.J.: Prentice-Hall, 1964.

Landers, Daniel, and Christina, Robert, eds. *Psychology of Motor Behavior and Sport*. Champaign, Ill.: Human Kinetics, 1977.

Loy, John W., Jr., and Kenyon, Gerald S., eds. *Sport, Culture and Society*. New York: Macmillan, 1969.

McIntosh, Peter C. *Sport in Society*. London: C. A. Watts, 1963.

Maheu, Rene. "Sport and Culture." *Journal of Health, Physical Education and Recreation* **34** (October 1963), pp. 30–32.

Martens, Rainer. "A Social Psychology of Physical Activity." *Quest* **14** (June 1970).

Morgan, William P., ed. *Contemporary Readings in Sport Psychology*. Springfield, Ill.: Charles C. Thomas, 1970.

Mosston, Muska. *Teaching Physical Education: From Command to Discovery*. Columbus, Ohio: Charles E. Merrill, 1966.

Oxendine, Joseph B. "Emotional Arousal and Motor Performance." *Quest* **13** (January 1970).

Resick, Matthew C.; Seidel, Beverly L.; and Mason, James. *Modern Administrative Practices in Physical Education and Athletics*. Reading, Mass.: Addison-Wesley, 1975.

Robb, Margaret D. *The Dynamics of Motor Skill Acquisition.* Englewood Cliffs, N.J.: Prentice-Hall, 1972.

Russell, William F. "Success Is a Journey." *Sports Illustrated* **32** (June 8, 1970).

Sage, George H. *Introduction to Motor Behavior.* Reading, Mass.: Addison-Wesley, 1971.

Schmidt, Richard A. *Motor Skills.* New York: Harper & Row, 1975.

Scott, M. Gladys. "The Contributions of Physical Activity to Psychological Development." In *Anthology of Contemporary Readings,* edited by H. S. Slusher and A. S. Lockhart. Dubuque, Iowa: W. C. Brown, 1970, pp. 129–144.

Singer, Robert N. *Motor Learning and Human Performance.* 2d ed. New York: Macmillan, 1975.

Snyder, Eldon E. "Aspects of Socialization in Sports and Physical Education." *Quest* **14** (June 1970).

Triplett, Norman. "The Dynamogenic Factors of Pacemaking and Competition." *American Journal of Psychology* **9** (1968), pp. 507–533.

Vanek, Miroslav, and Cratty, Bryant J. *Psychology and the Superior Athlete.* New York: Macmillan, 1970.

White, Cyril M. "Towards a Sociology of Physical Education and Sport, Some Theoretical Considerations." In *Anthology of Contemporary Readings,* edited by H. S. Slusher and A. S. Lockhart. Dubuque, Iowa: W. C. Brown, 1970.

Zajonc, Robert B. *Social Psychology: An Experimental Approach.* Belmont, Calif.: Wadsworth, 1966.

Part II
Pedagogical
Bases

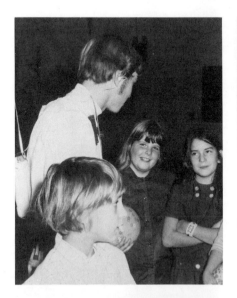

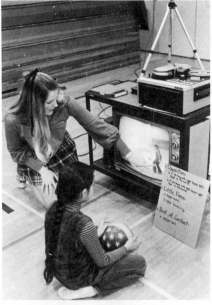

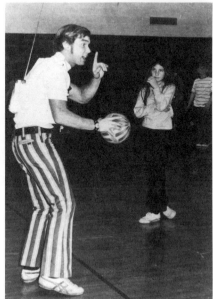

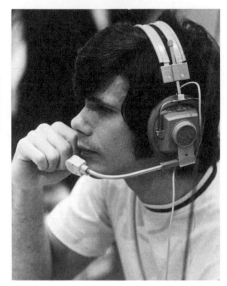

Modern pedagogy involves selection
and use of instructional media.

Chapter 7
Curriculum and the
School Program
in Physical
Education

Acceptance of all the traditional patterns of education
makes practitioners in any
field unresponsive to needed
changes and perpetuates
concepts and practices that
are no longer useful.

M. MACKENZIE MARLIN

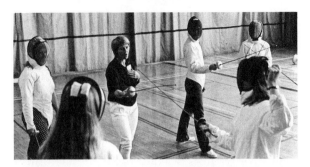

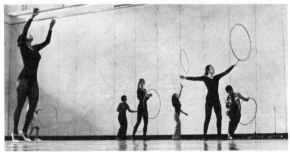

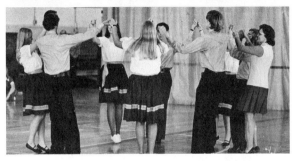

The modern school program in physical education
emphasizes a variety of activities.

P

EDAGOGY, the art and science of teaching, necessarily involves theoretical as well as practical considerations. It is probably safe to say, however, that just as physical educators have in the past been primarily concerned only with the practical, so too have pedagogical "theorists." In an attempt to acquaint the student who is just beginning his or her professional study in physical education with the fact that theoretical concepts ought to underlie practical pedagogical considerations, this chapter delineates some of the theoretical bases in the disciplines of education and physical education. Although the study of curriculum and its attendant development of a school program typically begins at the upper-division undergraduate or graduate level, an early exposure to curricular concepts and program building ought to motivate the student to recognize the need for further, more detailed study in this area.

Educational researchers traditionally have tended to concern themselves more with improving education than with understanding it. If curricular innovation is truly to be a catalyst for the improvement of education, then those who redesign curricula ought first to concern themselves with an understanding of curriculum theory with a view toward more nearly ensuring that the process and product of education are not confused. Johnson defines curriculum as a structured series of intended learning outcomes in which the results of instruction are anticipated, even prescribed.[1] Curriculum theorists, then, ought to be concerned with attainable learning experiences or ends, not with the means by which the results are accomplished nor even with a rationale for them. Curriculum theory is thus concerned with what it is intended that students learn (product) not with what it is intended that they do (process). Thus although curriculum is not a system per se, it may be conceptualized as the *output* of a "curriculum development system" and as the *input* into an "instructional system." Figure 7.1 is an example of a model which clearly depicts such a concept.

INTERRELATIONSHIPS OF AIMS, OBJECTIVES, AND CURRICULUM

Recent theorists are in substantial agreement that what can be learned can be divided into three categories of learning outcomes—cognitive affective, and psychomotor—and that aims and objectives can be formulated for each of them as a part of the *structured* series of intended learning outcomes. Since the learner is the focal point in both formal and informal situations, curricular concerns are not restricted to the classroom; such programs as intramurals are included as well. Regardless of the type of learning situation, attention must be centered on the results of instruction, and thus objectives in terms of behavioral outcomes must be defined. This approach is in almost direct opposition to the traditional

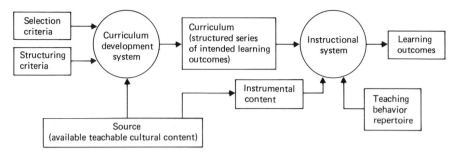

FIG. 7.1 **A model showing curriculum as an output of one system and an input of another. From Mauritz Johnson, Jr., "Definitions and Models in Curriculum Theory,"** *Educational Theory* **17 (April 1967), p. 132. Reprinted by permission.**

one in physical education, or any other subject, which prescribes instructional content as a means of achieving certain generalized objectives revolving around the acquisition of skill, knowledge, and attitudes. For example, the objective "to inculcate desirable social attitudes," though laudable, is so nebulous that it is perhaps overlooked more often than not by teachers as they plan and organize their instructional efforts. The objective "to assign to all squads the decision-making about the sharing of responsibility for setting up gymnastic equipment" is much more specific and much more easily evaluated, as well as designed to meet a "social" objective.

Regardless of the way objectives are stated, objectives per se are important if a true learning situation is to be structured. Inattention to the aims and purposes of education produces little more than a hodgepodge of "learning." Therefore, many educationists engage in philosophic discussions of what the aims of education in a particular society *ought* to be and of how best to proceed toward achieving them. The results of such study are manifested in curricular change.

The student who is preparing to become a teacher is constantly exposed to the terms *aims* and *objectives*. It is well, then, to formulate a working definition of them at the outset. An *aim* can be compared to the "impossible dream" of the Man of La Mancha or to Robert Browning's thought: "A man's reach should exceed his grasp, or what's a heaven for?" In other words, an aim is a statement of purpose so lofty as to be practically unattainable; whether it is reachable or not, however, there should be a ceaseless striving toward it. An *objective,* on the other hand, can be attained; it is but a rung on the ladder one climbs, a step at a time, in an all-out effort to achieve the purposes of education.

Any subject matter area in the total curriculum should contribute in some manner to the purposes of education and to the associated interpretation of experiences within its various realms. If it cannot, its place in the total educational perspective can properly be challenged. Therefore, the selection of and structuring of curricular materials within a subject area are based, to a significant extent, on how well they can meet the objectives and aims of the subject and thus, ultimately, of education. This inter-

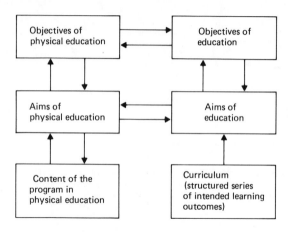

FIG. 7.2 Interrelationship of aims, objectives, and curriculum.

relationship is illustrated in Fig. 7.2. Note that no one phase can be an entity unto itself. Just as the content of the program in physical education contributes to the aims of education, so, too, the aims of education dictate curricular content.

Although statements of aims and objectives for the discipline of physical education and for its component parts are abundant in the professional literature, attempts at classifying educational goals are of but recent concern. Researchers in educational theory have found that most objectives can be covered by three domains, or classifications: (1) the *cognitive* domain, which encompasses those objectives which deal with intellectual emphases; (2) the *affective* domain, which includes objectives addressed to attitudes, appreciations, values, interests, and feelings; and (3) the *psychomotor* domain, which emphasizes motor skills and neuromuscular coordination.[2,3,4] The developed taxonomies (classifications) are of assistance to curriculum builders because they help to specify objectives "so that it becomes easier to plan learning experiences and prepare evaluative devices."[5]

TAXONOMIC MODELS, DOMAINS OF LEARNING

The basic structures of the taxonomic models in the three domains of learning are illustrated below so that the beginning student will have at least an initial awareness of them before enrolling in specific pedagogical courses.

A. Cognitive Domain (Knowledge, Intellectual Abilities)
The taxonomy of educational objectives in the cognitive domain as presented by Bloom and others is based on a hierarchical order, from concrete to abstract, of different classes of objectives.[6] It is assumed that the objectives proceed from the simplest intended behavior outcome to the most complex and that skills and abilities in the lowest classification are

essential for achievement in the next higher one and so on. A skeletal outline of the complete taxonomy follows:

Level One, Knowledge, including those behaviors which emphasize remembering of ideas, material, or phenomena:

1.00 Knowledge
    1.10 Knowledge of Specifics
    1.20 Knowledge of Ways and Means of Dealing with Specifics
    1.30 Knowledge of the Universals and Abstractions in a Field

Level Two, Comprehension, including those behaviors or responses which represent an understanding of the literal message of a communication:

2.00 Comprehension
    2.10 Translation
    2.20 Interpretation
    2.30 Extrapolation

Level Three, Application, including the ability to apply an abstraction correctly even though no method of solution is given. (Level Three is not subdivided into sequential steps.)

Level Four, Analysis, including the ability to breakdown learned material into its constituent parts and to detect the relationship of the parts:

4.00 Analysis
    4.10 Analysis of Elements
    4.20 Analysis of Relationships
    4.30 Analysis of Organizational Principles

Level Five, Synthesis, including the ability to put together constituent parts of the elements so as to form a whole:

5.00 Synthesis
    5.10 Production of a Unique Communication
    5.20 Production of a Plan, or Proposed Set of Operations
    5.30 Derivation of a Set of Abstract Relations

Level Six, Evaluation, including the ability to make value judgments about ideas, works, material, solutions, and the like:

6.00 Evaluation
    6.10 Judgments in Terms of Internal Evidence
    6.20 Judgments in Terms of External Criteria

B. Affective Domain (Attitudes, Values, Appreciations)
The taxonomy of objectives in the affective domain as described by Krathwohl, Bloom, and Masia is ordered in such a way that it delineates a process from a level of basic awareness to one of internalization.[7] The categories, as in the cognitive domain, are hierarchical in order, as follows:

Level One, Receiving (Attending), in which the learner is made aware of the existence of certain phenomena and stimuli:

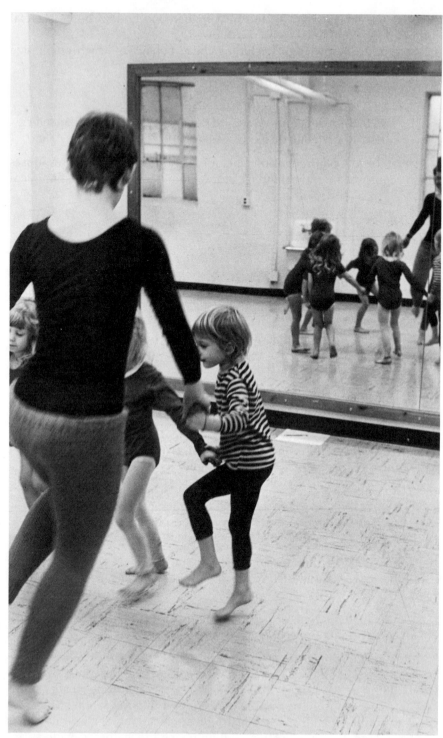

The affective domain (valuing, caring, sharing) must be encouraged early in the physical education of the child.

1.0 Receiving (Attending)
    1.1 Awareness
    1.2 Willingness to Receive
    1.3 Controlled or Selected Attention

Level Two, Responding, in which the learner goes beyond mere attending to *active* attending:

2.0 Responding
    2.1 Acquiescence in Responding
    2.2 Willingness to Respond
    2.3 Satisfaction in Response

Level Three, Valuing, in which the learner recognizes that a phenomenon or behavior has worth:

3.0 Valuing
    3.1 Acceptance of a Value
    3.2 Preference for a Value
    3.3 Commitment (Conviction)

Level Four, Organization, in which the learner begins to build a value system:

4.0 Organization
    4.1 Conceptualization of a Value
    4.2 Organization of a Value System

Level Five, Characterization by a Value or Value Complex, in which the learner, having internalized some kind of consistent value system, integrates his or her beliefs, attitudes and ideas into a total philosophy of life:

5.0 Characterization by A Value or Value Complex
    5.1 Generalized Set
    5.2 Characterization

C. Psychomotor Domain

Harrow's classification of observable motor behaviors outlined below is hierarchical from lowest to highest and is designed to assist educators in categorizing movement so that relevant educational goals can be structured.[8]

Level One, Reflex Movements, including such behavioral activity as flexion and extension:

1.00 Reflex Movements
    1.10 Segmental Reflexes
    1.20 Intersegmental Reflexes
    1.30 Suprasegmental Reflexes

Level Two, Fundamental Movements, including locomotor, nonloco-motor, and manipulative behaviors:

2.00 Basic-Fundamental Movements
    2.10 Locomotor Movements
    2.20 Nonlocomotor Movements
    2.30 Manipulative Movements

Level Three, Perceptual Abilities, including those abilities such as visual and tactile discrimination necessary for purposeful movement:

3.00 Perceptual Abilities
    3.10 Kinesthetic Discrimination
    3.20 Visual Discrimination
    3.30 Auditory Discrimination
    3.40 Tactile Discrimination
    3.50 Coordinated Discrimination

Level Four, Physical Abilities, including those components of physical fitness which are prerequisite to the formation and maintenance of highly skilled movement:

4.00 Physical Abilities
    4.10 Endurance
    4.20 Strength
    4.30 Flexibility
    4.40 Agility

Level Five, Skilled Movements, including activities, simple to complex, built upon the movement patterns classified in Level Two:

5.00 Skilled Movements
    5.10 Simple Adaptive Skill
    5.20 Compound Adaptive Skill
    5.30 Complex Adaptive Skill

Level Six, Nondiscursive Communication, including those bodily movements which act as forms of communication:

6.00 Nondiscursive Communication
    6.10 Expressive Movement
    6.20 Interpretive Movement

Several possible relationships between these taxonomies and the curriculum model shown in Fig. 7.1, page 95, should become evident as one recognizes that learning outcomes can be stated behaviorally in terms of the three domains of learning and that the attainment of them is more likely to be effectuated if attention is given to the depicted factors such as selection and structure of criteria and teaching behavior.

FACTORS INFLUENCING CURRICULAR CHANGE

The curriculum in physical education, as in any other subject, has undergone many and sometimes quite significant changes. Unlike the situation with some other subjects, however, the influences behind curricular revision in physical education have generally not come from within the school system itself or even from the state supervisors of physical education, whose chief function, at least theoretically, is the motivation of excellence. As an example, one need mention only the change in program content in physical education brought about by the Kraus-Weber report on the lack of physical fitness in American youth.

Although physical education was introduced into the school curriculum in the last part of the nineteenth century, until very recently there had been only one national-level effort, in 1929, aimed at developing guidelines for a comprehensive physical education curriculum. The guidelines published at that time were reexamined periodically, but no comprehensive attempt to evaluate them in light of contemporary educational philosophy under the aegis of national leadership was made until 1963, when a curriculum commission was established and funded by the American Association for Health, Physical Education and Recreation. This commission is charged with the task of examining curricula in physical education in light of current research in education, and it has reached agreement on the following points.

1. Current physical education curricula are a hodgepodge of activities with no pattern of consistency within them.

2. The resultant learnings from these curricula, at best, are not relevant to personal needs.

3. To be meaningful, physical education curricula must be constructed within a comprehensive conceptual framework.

4. The development of such a framework requires the diligent, long-term effort of many physical educators with diverse areas of specialization and expertise[9]

It seems safe to say that curricular changes in the past were based largely on practical problems, not theoretical concepts. Change so based can hardly be productive of the best learning. What are some of the factors, then, that ought to be considered if curricular change is to be more meaningful?

National influences run the gamut from professional guidance and direction given by national professional organizations to a determination of the social needs of American youth. Those needs must be examined by the professional before specific curricular avenues can be constructed. The federal government also constitutes a national influence through its subsidization of many school programs and its funding of research grants to study curricular problems. The vast American public, through what it values, must be reckoned with as a national influence as well. According to Leonard, it is indeed ironic that, in an age when sports are such an important spectacle in American society, physical education as a curricular area remains in the shadows in most schools.[10]

Greater attention to *empirical evidence* of the needs of students at various developmental stages is another factor influencing change. Whereas untested and unproven "theories" were used in the past as springboards for program change, research in education is sufficiently sophisticated today so that educational theorists are basing their explanation of specific student needs and their proposals for meeting these needs on verifiable evidence.

The *knowledge explosion,* dating back to 1957 and the launching of Sputnik, was an influencing factor of great magnitude. At the time, the public panicked and there was widespread criticism of education by lay people. Educators tended to overreact by emphasizing acquisition of knowledge to the exclusion of almost all other educational objectives. Nevertheless, the fact that knowledge increased tremendously and that a body of knowledge was delineated in physical education laid the groundwork for dramatic curricular change.

The *change in value systems* from one era to another cannot help being influential in changing curricular concepts. Educators are wrestling with the philosophic question of what values *ought* to be stressed in American society. Differing philosophic viewpoints produce different value continua, but there needs to be at least basic agreement on a theoretical framework of values from which curriculum makers can construct models for action.

Legal decisions in reference to education and physical education have had tremendous impacts on school programs. On occasion, the courts mandate the abolishment of certain regulations (for example, dress codes determined to be too restrictive). State legislatures, based on proposals from state boards of education, impose curricular requirements in terms of both subject matter and amounts of credit. The most recent example of a legal mandate of great magnitude is Title IX, that portion of the Equal Rights Amendment which deals with sex discrimination. The manifestation of this piece of legislation in terms of programming, budgeting, and scheduling of facilities is far-reaching.

A listing of the factors cited above, though by no means exhaustive, would be flexible enough to permit a more sophisticated delineation of factors which influence curricular change within its framework. For example, greater attention to empirical evidence can provide answers to questions revolving around such matters as personality needs of children and abilities of children to learn specific content at certain developmental stages.

IMPLICATIONS FOR PHYSICAL EDUCATION

Nearly all contemporary thinking about the process of curriculum development and change revolves around conceptual systems and theoretical models. According to Goodlad, a *conceptual system* identifies: (1) major questions that need to be answered in curriculum development, (2) elements that bind those questions into some kind of system, (3) subordinate questions, and (4) sources of data that can be used to answer the initial questions.[11] On the other hand, a *theoretical model* is "a visual, diagrammatic or three-dimensional representation of the interlocking elements of a conceptual system."[12]

Curriculum theorists in physical education are no exception to this "new breed" of educationists, and most of the recent literature in physical education curriculum construction also follows a "conceptual system" and "theoretical model" approach.

Perhaps the single most cogent treatment of the implications of curriculum theory for physical education is that by Jewett. The five implications she discusses and analyzes are summarized below:

1. The concept approach to curriculum development in physical education is most productive of significant improvement. Its potential, therefore, should be vigorously and scientifically pursued.
2. The problem of defining physical education and delineating its body of knowledge must be attacked with renewed vigor.
3. An acceptable conceptual (theoretical) model for the curriculum in physical education must be constructed. Existing models, both within and without the discipline of physical education, are not necessarily the most satisfactory ones.
4. Statements of objectives for physical education curricula must be drastically improved. Traditional statements are far too generalized; descriptions of specific behavioral outcomes are needed.
5. The problems of professional specialization within the discipline of physical education need to be analyzed more objectively. Therefore graduate study of curriculum must be encouraged as much as research in exercise physiology, sociology and psychology of sports, and other more commonly accepted areas.[13]

Attempts at curriculum renovation have blossomed in the past few years. Even though sometimes quite dramatic, much of this activity has been fragmented and nonproductive. Attention should be directed, then, toward a more global concept of curriculum in order to ensure true progress toward an effective educational system. Direction signals cannot be more distinctly charted, however, until the study of curriculum becomes one of recognized importance and until special curricular research competencies are developed and nurtured among physical education scholars. Genuine progress is being made; yet much remains to be done.

THE SCHOOL PROGRAM IN PHYSICAL EDUCATION

Physical education today is characterized by exciting, dramatic, and almost constant changes. The PEPI (Physical Education Public Information) proj-

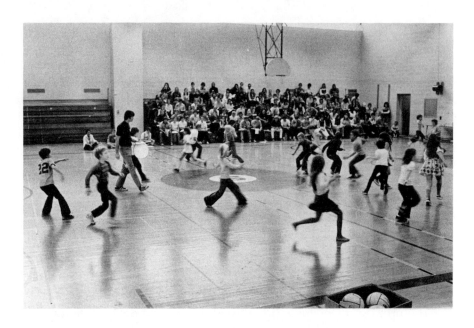

In-service workshops are a means of continuing professional growth.

ect and its attention to the "new physical education" is but one example of this. It can be said with more than a fair degree of accuracy, however, that the "typical" school program in physical education is not difficult to describe. (Read again Leonard's characterization of such a program in Chapter 1). As a matter of fact, the former Superintendent of Schools of the state of California quite accurately stated that the physical education class in most high schools is characterized by taking attendance, checking out a bunch of balls to a bunch of kids, and telling them to play the game.[14] Any criticism by the authors of current programs is not meant to disparage the teachers or the schools; our purpose is rather to draw attention to the great need for change.

AIMS AND OBJECTIVES

Traditionally, physical education has attempted to be all things to all people. Almost regardless of stated educational objectives, physical educators industriously tried to prove how they could teach toward them. In fact, physical education was so involved in being "educational" that it seemed to overlook what its unique concerns *ought* to be. As pointed out in the last chapter, this situation is changing as theorists wrestle with curricular concepts. We can hope, as the theorists construct conceptual curricula, that the practitioners will change teaching procedures to keep pace. A recent issue of *Quest* deals exclusively and cogently with this concern.[15]

There is rather strong agreement today that the focus of the discipline of physical education is human movement. It therefore seems logical that the aim of this area of study is to teach students to use their bodies efficiently and effectively in all movement patterns because they have a cognitive understanding of movement, as well as an affective appreciation of the value of purposeful movement.

Although objectives can be stated in many different ways, there is a definite trend today toward stating them as behavioral outcomes. Beginning professional students in physical education will be introduced further to these various ways when they are exposed to methodology and pedagogy. Statements of objectives can be found in almost any textbook, any syllabus, or any course of study. One of the criticisms leveled against writers of objectives is that such statements are generally elusive, if not illusory, and therefore of little value to the teacher. Esbensen says that a well-stated objective needs to define what a students will be able to do under what conditions and to what extent.[16]

1. "The student should have an adequate comprehension of the principles of movement." No one would quarrel with this statement, but it does not tell us what the student should be able to *do* as a result of this "comprehension," nor does it define the *condition* of "adequate."

2. "The student should be able to use the vocabulary of basic movement so that he or she can act appropriately to verbal stimuli." This statement defines a *condition* of "verbal stimuli," but it does not mention to what *extent* the child should be able to use movement vocabulary.

3. "The student should be able to traverse within ten seconds a twenty-foot obstacle course while manipulating a ball." This statement delineates performance, extent, and a condition.

4. "Children need to learn to accept responsibility." This statement, though no doubt true, is not expressed in terms of a behavioral outcome, nor does it meet any of Esbensen's criteria.

Regardless of the manner in which objectives are stated, the following are most often properly considered to be physical education objectives.

1. *Organic development, or physical fitness.* Many physical educators describe this objective as being the most important one. Whether one agrees or not, it cannot be denied that physical education is the only school program concerned with the development of strength, endurance, and other attributes of physical fitness.

2. *Skill development.* Neuromuscular coordination and the development and refinement of movement and activity skills are certainly also unique to physical education.

3. *Emotional health.* One who learns specific activity skills well so that he or she can engage in some of the "lifetime sports" during leisure time is more apt to be able to cope with the pressures of everyday living.

4. *Mental development.* Awareness and understanding of the principles of movement constitute but one example of how physical education can contribute to the "mental development" of the child.

5. *Social development.* Desirable attitudes, such as courage, sharing, fair play, and concern for others, can be fostered in a properly conducted program of physical education.

A great many educational theorists today propose that objectives for the students, as expressed by them, should also be considered in any planning for instruction. Such objectives typically include the following.

1. To develop a positive self-concept.
2. To be accepted as a member of a group or team.
3. To increase enjoyment in sports participation through skill refinement.
4. To relax and forget study pressures.

All of the objectives above are appropriate to physical education, and the manner in which the individual instructor deals with them will no doubt be determined by his or her value system. Figure 7.3 shows a well-known ordered and logical arrangement of objectives which can be related without too much difficulty to the curriculum model on p. 95.[17] Note that Bookwalter's hierarchy follows rather closely those concepts of aims and objectives previously discussed. The ultimate aim is philosophic, and its complete attainment is at best difficult. The objectives range from remote (general) to immediate (specific), and they are finally expressed as outcomes (behavioral goals).

It is doubtful that any attempt to arranging a hierarchy of objectives, whether from the instructor's or from the student's point of view, would be entirely acceptable. Thus the importance of the value judgment underlying educational concerns is apparent. According to Brackenbury, educators must turn to philosophers for help in determining those values important in a democratic society.[18] Unfortunately, philosophers seem to have abrogated that responsibility, and thus there is confusion about desired goals for education. Philosophy and education must work together and become mutually reconstructive if education is to become more meaningful.[19]

EXAMPLES OF CURRICULUM IN PHYSICAL EDUCATION

Although the curriculum includes more than the formal course of study, when one considers the program of activities in a particular subject, one is usually thinking in terms of curriculum.

La Porte's classic, *Physical Education Curriculum,* presents a "carefully graded curriculum" which serves two purposes: (1) to set standards in physical education, and (2) to unify programs so that children can transfer from school to school without losing continuity in instruction.[20] This

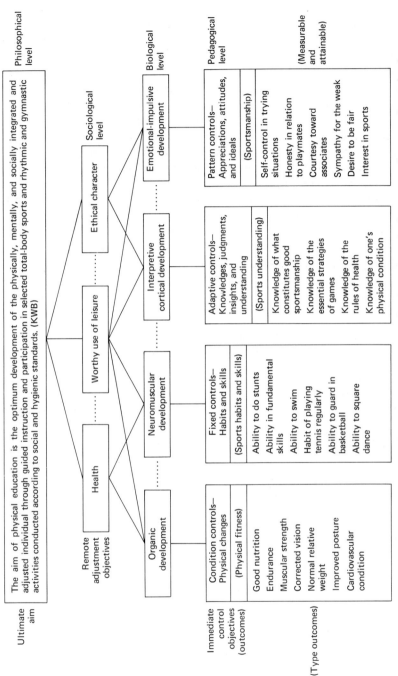

FIG. 7.3 **The purposes of physical education.** From K. W. Bookwalter, *Physical Education in the Secondary Schools* (Washington, D.C., 1964), The Center for Applied Research in Education, Inc. **Reprinted by permission.**

treatise, originally published in 1937, has undergone several revisions, the latest by Cooper in 1968. It is not surprising that a study attempting to achieve the purposes stated above tends to be overstructured. Although the authors state that the suggested percentages of time for particular types of activity are only approximate and that the listed activities are merely samplings, there are invariably some teachers and supervisors who must "go by the book." Under such circumstances, the program immediately loses sight of its product, the individual child. Tables 7.1, 7.2, and 7.3 are reproductions of the sample programs advocated by La Porte and his associates. So long as the professional student uses them in the manner intended, they can be beneficial in program planning.

As mentioned before, the greatest drawback in listing activities in tabular form, along with suggested time allotments for each, is the apparent lack of concern for the learner. Critics of education today constantly decry the "dehumanizing" process that is carried on in "joyless" schools.[21] The trend toward movement education, as discussed in Chapter 8, along with its attendant methodology, represents a significant attempt to make the learner the core of the educative process. Mosston's plea for changing teaching techniques in physical education so that the

Table 7.1   Sample Program for the Primary Level (Grades 1–3)

1. *Fundamental Movements* 20%
   Locomotor: walking, running, skipping, galloping, whirling, swaying.
   Axial: swinging, sustaining, etc.
2. *Rhythmic Activities* (could be combined with locomotor activities if music accompaniment is used): 20%
   Farmer in the Dell, Looby Loo, Mulberry Bush, Chimes of Dunkirk, Old Roger Is Dead, The Swing, Carrousel, Jolly Is the Miller, Oats, peas, beans, etc.
3. *Games* 30%
   Simple chasing games such as cat and mice, Jack be nimble, squirrel in trees, cat and rat, hound and rabbit, midnight, lame fox and chickens, etc.
   Athletic games such as boundary ball, hand polo, kick ball, bound ball.
4. *Self-Testing Activities* 30%
   Duck walk, rabbit hop, human rocker, crab walk, forward roll, frog hand stand, etc.
5. *Relays* (part of games and/or self-testing section)

   Total 100%

   Swimming should be offered here if a pool is available.

Note: Description of above typical activities will be found in most game books and elementary school manuals. The activities listed are merely samplings.

The time allotments indicated in percentages are approximate, merely to indicate the relative importance. These will vary somewhat with grade—relays receiving emphasis from the second grade on, and athletic games from the third grade on. In many cases the activities included under the several headings will be selected from the subject matter of a given *unit of work* or *center of interest* around which the entire program of a given grade may be centered. It is very important that the physical education activities be integrated with the rest of the program of this level.

William Ralph La Porte, *The Physical Education Curriculum*, revised by John M. Cooper, Indiana University (Los Angeles: College Book Store, 1968), p. 29.

Table 7.2 Sample Program for the Elementary Level (Grades 4–6)

1. *Games* 50%
   Athletic games
      Basketball type: captain ball, captain basketball, corner ball, line basketball, nine-court basketball, newcomb, six-court basketball, six-hole basketball, quadruple dodge ball.
      Softball type: bombardment, bat ball, circle strike, end ball, fongo, hit pin baseball, long ball, one and two old cat, triangle ball, and work up.
      Soccer type: advancement, circle soccer, corner kick ball, field ball, kick ball, punt back, rotation soccer, simplified soccer, soccer dodge ball, and soccer keep away.
      Volleyball type: bound ball, feather ball, net ball, schoolroom volleyball and sponge ball.
   Chasing games
      Bears and cattle, circle chase, gathering sticks, two and three deep, catch of fish, last man, pom pom pullaway, all stand, club snatch, cross tag, dare base, duck on a rock, prisoner's base, etc.
2. *Rhythmical Activities* 20%
   Broom dance, Dutch couple dance, Pop goes the Weasel, Bleking, Virginia Reel, Sellengers Round, Ace of Diamonds, Gustaf's Skoal, Seven Jumps, Norwegian Mountain March, Lottie Is Dead, etc.
3. *Self-Testing* 30%
   Events: Batting for accuracy, base running, baseball throw for accuracy, basketball pass for accuracy—for goal—for distance, pull up, push up, broad jump, high jump, soccer kick for goal—distance, etc.
   Stunts: Head stand, forward roll, backward roll, cartwheel, heel click, wooden man, jump the stick, Indian wrestle, Eskimo roll, front foot flip, knee and toe wrestle, hand wrestle, knee spring elephant walk, triple roll, etc.
4. *Relays* (Part of games and/or self-testing sections)
   Arch ball relay, hopping relay, stunt relays, all-up Indian club relay, over and under relay, shuttle relay, stride ball relay, skin the snake relay, etc.
5. *Inclement Weather Activities* (Games that may be conducted in the classroom.)

   Total 100%

Note: Descriptions of the above typical activities can be found in most game books and elementary school manuals. The activities listed are merely samplings.

The time allotments in percentages are approximate, to suggest relative importance. The selection of activities as in the primary level should be adapted to the *center of interest or culture area* being studied at the time in a given grade. It is suggested that the self-testing events be practiced as an integral part of the corresponding game and that many of the relays be composed of elements of the same game. Tumbling stunts should be kept very simple, and rhythmical activities should include good variety. In all activities emphasis should be placed on proper *body mechanics,* and on *fundamental skills* of running, jumping, throwing, catching, striking, kicking, etc.

William Ralph La Porte, *The Physical Education Curriculum,* revised by John M. Cooper, Indiana University (Los Angeles: College Book Store, 1968), p. 30.

individual learner is not subjugated to the group is being heard by more and more concerned teachers of physical education.[22]

The bias of the authors that physical education is an academic discipline would seem to demand of any model of curriculum in physical education that it be based on a conceptual rather than a time/activity approach. As discussed in Chapter 1, the focus of the discipline of physi-

Table 7.3 Sample Program for the Junior High School (Grades 7–9) and Senior High School (Grades 10–12)

	Boys Weeks	Girls Weeks	Boys Weeks	Girls Weeks
1. *Survival and Water Safety* Swimming — Diving — Lifesaving	18	18	12	12
2. *Dancing and Rhythms* Folk — Square — Social — Modern (Girls)	12	18	12	18
3. *Team Sports* a) *Court and Diamond Games* Volleyball — Softball — Basketball — 2-Court Basketball (Junior High Girls)	18	18	12	12
b) *Field Sports* Soccer — Speedball — Touch Football (Boys) — Fieldball (Junior High Girls) — Field Hockey (Senior High Girls)	18	12	18	12
4. *Tumbling Gymnastics* Tumbling — Pyramids — Apparatus — Relays — Stunts — Body Mechanics and Body Building — Endurance and Strength	12	12	12	12
5. *Individual and Dual Sports* a) Tennis — Badminton — Handball or Golf or Archery	12	12	30*	30*
b) *Additional Sports and Activities* selected from the following list: Boating and Canoeing — Bowling — Bowling — Hiking and Camping — Horseshoes — Fencing — Fly and Bait Casting — Paddle Tennis — Riding — Skating — Snowshoeing — Squash — Table Tennis — Trampoline — Weight Training — Outdoor Education — Wrestling; or, devote more time to dual activities listed under (a) but many should be in co-educational activities	18	18	12	12
	Total of 108 Weeks		Total of 108 Weeks	

*Some choice permitted where feasible.

Notes to Table 7.3

The time allotments are approximate in terms of relative values, and are subject to minor adjustment. They are listed in terms of weeks. A given activity can be concentrated in one year with a specific number of weeks or it may be split between two of the three years or distributed equally among the three years according to preference of a given school. If desired, it is possible to schedule the activities to fit seasonal sports.

It is understood that this schedule is for class instruction purposes, to be supplemented by an opportunity for extensive intramural participation by all students. Where this extra laboratory period is not available, the last third or fourth part of the regular class period should be devoted to enthusiastic participation in the activity or game being studied. In any case, sufficient participation should be given in the class period to assure adequate motivation and appreciation of the game as a unified whole.

It is recommended that in connection with all activities, basic instruction and guidance be given in fundamental body mechanics, the efficient use of the body as a coordinated unit. The most effective instruction in the proper handling of the body probably comes from good example plus repeated cautioning on how to hold and to use the body in a variety of situations—functional posture. This involves the development of both protective skills and expressive skills.

It is recommended that each activity be given continuously for at least six weeks, at the senior high level. This would mean that the class instruction in a given activity such as basketball would appear in only one of the three years of the senior high. A student should have opportunity, however, for additional participation in the intramural program or the interschool team program.

William Ralph La Porte, The Physical Education Curriculum, revised by John M. Cooper, Indiana University (Los Angeles: College Book Store, 1968), pp 31–32.

cal education is human movement. The concept of human movement is necessarily much broader than specific sports or activities as shown in Tables 7.4 and 7.5. Notice that each triangular dimension overlaps the others and that the entire program is ostensibly less highly structured than that advocated by La Porte. Such a conceptual approach has been criticized on at least two counts. Some physical educators decry that this approach to human movement education, while perhaps beneficial at the lower grades level, neglects specialized sports skills. This fear ought to be allayed by an examination of Table 7.5 which plots a progression from foundational to specialized movement experiences. In addition, some physical educators seem willing to accept the conceptual approach at the elementary school level but they doubt its effectiveness at the higher levels of education. The perusal of a recent book, Sports Skills: A Conceptual Approach to Meaningful Movement,[23] ought to allay these doubts as well.

The different tables in this chapter may confuse the student since they seem to indicate a lack of consensus among curriculum makers as to exactly what should be included in a program of activities at a particular level. Quite so! Indeed, it would be unrealistic to expect complete agreement on such a complex topic, because each teacher, as an individual, has a philosophy of physical education uniquely his or her own. For example, note that Table 7.1 indicates that children in grade 1–3 should receive approximately 20 percent of their total physical education instructional time in rhythmic activities, and the table lists several examples of singing games, such as "Farmer in the Dell" and "Looby Loo." However, the instructor who teaches from the movement education perspective (see Chapter 5) would first proclaim that 20 percent of the total instructional time is far too little for rhythms at the primary level, and would also decry the lack of opportunity for children to be creative in such a structured activity as "Farmer in the Dell." Conversely, the instructor who is not movement-education oriented is not likely to be easily convinced that the approach shown in Tables 7.4 and 7.5 allows sufficient time to

Table 7.4 Model of Developmental Phases Related to Movement Experiences

	Early Phase	Subsequent Phase	Later Phase	Late Phase
	Awareness	Fundamental Skills	Specialized Skills	Movement (Skill) Specialization
	Self: body parts movement potential Kinesthesia Environment: changes, limitations, possibilities	Proficiency Appropriate use of body parts. Combinations of movement.	Effective combinations of movement elements and fundamental motor skills. Quality and purpose. Movement commonalities in selected specialized skills	Utilization of related components of previous phases. Skill in perception of intra and interdisciplinary relationships.
	Self-Confidence Movement control Achievement Acceptance	Self-Understanding Differentiation between importance of self and group. Desire and ability to control movement. Body structure and movement potential.	Self-Evaluation Critical evaluation of movement. Body potential for achieving excellence in specific form Acceptance. Realistic view of achievement.	Self-Actualization Establishing own value system. Discrete quality of self-discipline. Acceptance of self, capacities, worth.
	Habits of Thought Movement vocabulary Kinesthetic, verbal selection of appropriate movements to solve problems	Habits of Thought Significance of proficiency. Relationship of movement results to principles of human movement. Importance of effective group action. Relationship between movement elements, body, and fundamental motor skills.	Habits of Thought Decision making—selection of appropriate movement combinations, strategy applied through movement contributes to control of self and environment; to feeling of worth and power over self. Valuing movement. Relationship of mechanical laws of motion to principles of human movement.	Habits of Thought Continuous modification and application of ideas for productive change.

Developmental Phases

Movement Experiences

Courtesy of Naomi Allenbaugh, Emeritus Professor of Physical Education, the Ohio State University.

Table 7.5 Model for Movement Experiences Foundational to Specialized

Physical Education Content — Knowledge and Skills

Movement Tasks Based on content involving:	*Fundamental Motor Skill Tasks* Designed for study of:	*Specialized Motor Skills Tasks* Designed for study of:	*Specialization in Selected Activity Skills* Toward "championship" performance:
1. Movement elements space, force, time, flow, and their dimensions	3. Locomotor skills 4. Nonlocomotor skills 5. Manipulative skills and the	Sequences of movement using fundamental motor skills and movement elements designed to achieve a specific purpose in a particular activity:	High level of movement proficiency in skill sequences. Use of movement commonalities; application of movement patterns, space-force-time factors, strategies, etc.
2. Body focus Relationships Leads Support Transfer of weight Control	6. Principles of Human Movement (Follow through) (Opposition) (Objective Focus) (Total Assembly)	Forms of More Complex Traditional Activities: games, sports, dance, gymnastics, aquatics	*Habits of Thought* Application of knowledge and Kinesthesia (feedback) for Movement evaluation and improvement.
Simple Form: Traditional Activities— games, dance, gymnastics, aquatics, utilizing knowledges and skills derived from 1 and 2 above	*Modified Forms:* Traditional Activities— games, dance, gymnastics, aquatics, utilizing knowledges and skills derived from 1, 2, 3, 4, 5, 6	*Mechanical Laws of Motion* Gravity Leverage Equilibrium Force Rebound Spin	Decision making.

Courtesy of Naomi Allenbaugh, Emeritus Professor of Physical Education, the Ohio State University.

develop specialized sports skills. Thus it once again becomes apparent that attention to philosophic bases underlying activity programs is of prime importance.

SUMMARY

Education today professes a belief in individual expression, self-control, and self-actualization. The school program in physical education will more nearly embrace these concepts—in theory as well as in practice—as physical educators pay more attention to the delineation of objectives based on individual needs, the subsequent formulation of programs which will best meet these objectives, and the import of curriculum theory.

STUDENT PROJECTS

1. With the class divided into three sections, research and report on the three taxonomies of objectives listed. Select a specific activity, write objectives for it in terms of behavioral outcomes, and classify them according to the taxonomies.
2. Classify the statements in Tables 7.4 and 7.5 according to the domains of learning.
3. Conduct an informal survey among a sampling of students living in your residence hall to determine the program of activities they had in their high school physical education programs. Include information on the approximate amount of time spent in each activity.
4. Review the theoretical models in some of the selected references (e.g., Galloway, Jewett, Vogel). Are they similar conceptually? In what ways are they dissimilar?

GLOSSARY OF TERMS

Curricuum   A structured series of intended learning outcomes. It can be formal or informal, in-class or extra-class.

Aim   A philosophic statement of an educational goal which is purposely remote.

Objective   A less remote statement of an educational goal. Objectives are usually characterized as "general" (broad in scope) or "specific" (limited in scope).

Taxonomy of objectives   A classification of objectives so that those similar in nature are grouped together under a common heading.

Cognitive domain   Those objectives which deal with intellectual emphases.

Affective domain   Those objectives which deal with attitudes, appreciations, feelings, and values.

Psychomotor domain Those objectives which deal with motor skills and neuromuscular coordination.

Concept A key idea which is complete and therefore meaningful to the learner.

Model A visual representation of a concept.

Pedagogy The art and science of teaching.

Philosophy of education An area of systematic study which attempts to guide educational theory and practice.

Behavioral outcomes Objectives or goals for any course of study expressed in terms of desired behavior.

Review all the terms listed for Chapter 3.

REFERENCES

1. Mauritz Johnson, Jr., "Definitions and Models in Curriculum Theory," *Educational Theory* **17** (April 1967), 127–140.

2. Benjamin S. Bloom, ed., *Taxonomy of Educational Objectives, Handbook I: Cognitive Domain* (New York: David McKay, 1956).

3. David R. Krathwohl, Benjamin S. Bloom, and Bertram Masia, *Taxonomy of Educational Objectives. Handbook II: Affective Domain* (New York: David McKay, 1964).

4. Anita J. Harrow, *A Taxonomy of the Psychomotor Domain* (New York: David McKay, 1972).

5. Bloom, p. 2.

6. Ibid., pp. 201–207.

7. Krathwohl, Bloom, and Masia, p. 95.

8. Harrow, pp. 1–2.

9. Anita Aldrich, *Cooperative Development of Design for Long-Term Research Project Directed Toward the Identification and Evaluation of a Conceptual Framework for the Curriculum in Physical Education, Grades K-16* (Washington: American Association for Health, Physical Education and Recreation, 1967), pp. 1–2.

10. George Leonard, "Why Johnny Can't Run," *The Atlantic*, (August 1975), 55–60.

11. John I. Goodlad, "Curriculum: The State of the Field," *Review of Educational Research* **30** (June 1960), pp. 195–196.

12. Elizabeth C. Wilson, "A Model for Action," in *Rational Planning in Curriculum and Instruction* (Washington: National Education Association, 1967), p. 165.

13. Ann E. Jewett, "Implications from Curriculum Theory for Physical Education," *The Academy Papers* **2** (October 1968), pp. 10–18.

14. Max L. Rafferty, Jr., "A Critical Look at Physical Education," *California Journal of Secondary Education* **33** (January 1958), p. 32.

15. "Educational Changes in the Teaching of Physical Education," *Quest* **15** (January 1971).

16. Thorwald Esbensen, "Writing Educational Objectives," *Phi Delta Kappan* **48** (January 1967), pp. 246–247.

17. Karl W. Bookwalter, *Physical Education in the Secondary Schools* (Washington: Center for Applied Research in Education, 1964), p. 13.

18. Robert L. Brackenbury, "Guidelines to Help Schools Formulate and Validate Objectives," in *Rational Planning in Curriculum and Instruction* (Washington: National Education Association, 1967), pp. 89–108.

19. Charles J. Brauner and Hobert W. Burns, *Problems in Education and Philosophy* (Englewood Cliffs, N.J.: Prentice-Hall, 1965), p. 20.

20. William Ralph La Porte (revised by John M. Cooper, Indiana University), *The Physical Education Curriculum* (Los Angeles: College Book Store, 1968).

21. Charles Silberman, *Crisis in the Classroom* (New York: Random House, 1970).

22. Muska Mosston, *Teaching Physical Education: From Command to Discovery* (Columbus, Ohio: Charles E. Merrill, 1966).

23. Beverly L. Seidel et al. *Sports Skills: A Conceptual Approach to Meaningful Movement.* Dubuque, Iowa: W. C. Brown, 1975.

SELECTED READINGS

Alley, Louis E. "Research and the Curriculum in Physical Education." In *Research Methods in Health, Physical and Recreation.* 2d ed. Washington: American Association for Health, Physical Education and Recreation, 1959.

Bloom, Benjamin S., ed. *Taxonomy of Educational Objectives. Handbook I: Cognitive Domain.* New York: David McKay, 1956.

Bookwalter, Karl W. *Physical Education in Secondary Schools.* Washington: Center for Applied Research in Education, 1964.

Brackenbury, Robert L. "Guidelines to Help Schools Formulate and Validate Objectives." In *Rational Planning in Curriculum and Instruction.* Washington: National Education Association, 1967.

Bruner, Charles J., and Burns, Hobert W. *Problems in Education and Philosophy.* Englewood Cliffs, N.J.: Prentice-Hall, 1965.

Brown, Camille, and Cassidy, Rosalind. *Theory in Physical Education.* Philadelphia: Lea & Febiger, 1963.

Clein, Marvin, and Stone, William J. "Physical Education and the Classification of Educational Objectives: Psychomotor Domain." *Physical Educator* **27** (March 1970), pp. 34–35.

Conner, Forrest E., and Ellena, William J., eds. *Curriculum Handbook for School Administrators.* Washington: American Association of School Administrators, 1967.

Cowell, Charles C., and Hazelton, Helen. *Curriculum Designs in Physical Education.* Englewood Cliffs, N.J.: Prentice-Hall, 1959.

"Educational Change in the Teaching of Physical Education." *Quest* **15** (January 1971).

Esbensen, Thorwald. "Writing Educational Objectives." *Phi Delta Kappan* **48** (January 1967).

Galloway, Jane P. "A Conceptual Approach for Determining Patterns of Professional Preparation for Women in Health and Physical Education." Ed. D. diss. University of North Carolina, Greensboro, 1969.

Goodlad, John I., "Curriculum: The State of the Field." *Review Educational Research* **30** (June 1960).

Harrow, Anita J. *A Taxonomy of the Psychomotor Domain.* New York: David McKay, 1972.

Jewett, Ann E. "Implications from Curriculum Theory for Physical Education." *The Academy Papers* **2** (October 1968).

Johnson, Mauritz, Jr. "Definitions and Models in Curriculum Theory." *Educational Theory* **17** (April 1967), pp. 127–140.

Krathwohl, David R.; Bloom, Benjamin S.; and Masia, Bertram. *Taxonomy of Educational Objectives. Handbook II: Affective Domain.* New York: David McKay, 1964.

La Porte, William Ralph. *The Physical Education Curriculum,* Los Angeles: College Book Store, 1968.

Leonard, George. "Why Johnny Can't Run." *The Atlantic* (August 1975), pp. 55–60.

MacKenzie, Marlin M. *Toward a New Curriculum in Physical Education.* McGraw-Hill, 1969.

Mager, Robert F. *Preparation Objectives for Programmed Instruction.* San Francisco: Fearon Press, 1962.

Marconnit, George D., and Short, Edmund C., eds. *Contemporary Thought in Public School Curriculum.* Dubuque, Iowa: W. C. Brown, 1968.

Mosston, Muska. *Teaching Physical Education: From Command to Discovery.* Columbus, Ohio: Charles E. Merrill, 1966.

National Education Association, Center for the Study of Instruction. "Curriculum for People." *Today's Education* **60** (February 1971), pp. 42–44.

National Education Association, Center for the Study of Instruction. *Rational Planning in Curriculum and Instruction.* Washington: National Education Association, 1967.

Nixon, John E., and Jewett, Ann E. *Physical Education Curriculum.* New York: Ronald Press, 1964.

Pelton, Barry C. *New Curriculum Perspectives.* Dubuque, Iowa: W. C. Brown, 1970.

Phillips, James A., Jr. "General Trends in Curriculum Development Today." *The Ohio High School Athlete* (May 1968), pp. 207–209.

Rafferty, Max L., Jr. "A Critical Look at Physical Education." *California Journal of Secondary Education* **33** (January 1958).

Seidel, Beverly L. et al. *Sports Skills: A Conceptual Approach to Meaningful Movement.* Dubuque: W. C. Brown Co., 1975.

Silberman, Charles. *Crisis in the Classroom.* New York: Random House 1970.

Taba, Hilda. *Curriculum Development: Theory and Practice.* New York: Harcourt, Brace and World, 1962.

Vogel, Paul. "Battle Creek Education Curriculum Project." *Journal of Health, Physical Education and Recreation* (September 1969), pp. 25–29.

Wilson, Elizabeth C. "A Model for Action." *Rational Planning in Curriculum and Instruction.* Washington: National Education Association, 1967.

Chapter 8
Movement
Education

Every new movement or
manifestation of human activity, when unfamiliar to
people's minds, is sure to be
misrepresented and misun-
derstood.

EDWARD CARPENTER

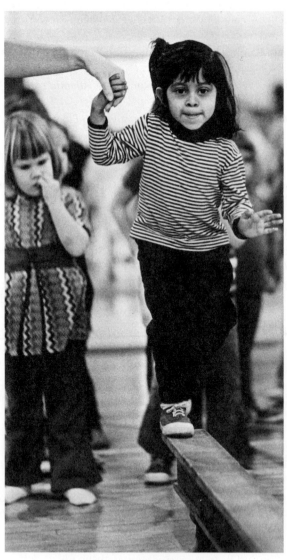

Children accept new movement
patterns as a challenge.

M

OVEMENT education has perhaps been the most noteworthy trend in physical education in the United States in the past decade, if not in this century. And as suggested in the quotation on the preceding page it has been widely misrepresented and just as widely misundertood. The quandary regarding the "movement movement" is due to several factors. Since the methodology of movement education consists largely of problem-solving and guided discovery, many critics of the movement see in it a regression to the throw-the-ball-out-and-let-them-go-at-it type of "instruction" that has been all too prevalent in the field. Some of the confusion is due to semantics, some to ignorance of the movement, some to lack of agreement among those who profess to be experts in the area, and some to the fact that overly enthusiastic advocates have made unwarranted claims for movement education and have thereby isolated potential supporters who prefer more tangible proof before they embrace what may be just another fad. What follows is an attempt to describe objectively the history of movement education as a curriculum—its purposes, its program, its justification, and its probable future.

HISTORY

Movement education received an impetus in Great Britain in the 1940s and earlier, when there arose a new conception of human movement, revolving at least partially around the work of Rudolf Laban, a dancer and choreographer, and his theory of movement analysis based on *what* moves, *how* it moves, *where* it moves, and what the relationship of the movement with other moving and nonmoving factors is. *Educational gymnastics,* the term used in the British movement, has as its objective the teaching of efficient body movement through a skillful combination of movements in relation to space, force, time, and flow, the commonly accepted *elements of movement.*[1] The program is characterized by a focus on conceptual content, movement exploration, great quantities of equipment, creative teaching, and less structured lessons. In addition to fostering skill in managing the body in a variety of circumstances, the program stresses cognitive aspects of movement since the body cannot be trained in a vacuum. The affective domain also receives emphasis as youngsters experience in and through movement a concern for others, a growing sense of confidence with an attendant lessening of self-consciousness, and an awareness of pleasureful activity as skill levels increase. Thus the three classifications of educational objectives, as discussed in Chapter 3, can be met in a program of movement education. As more and more American teachers of physical education observed these British gymnastics lessons, noting the methodology employed and the good results obtained, they became extremely interested in exploration as a

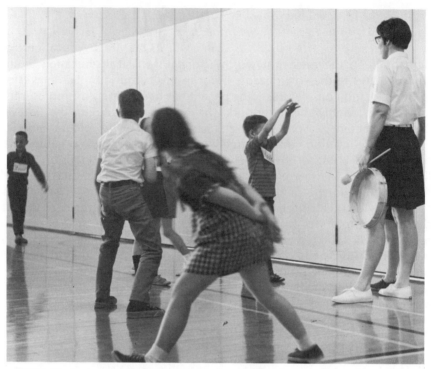

Children learn to move; children move to learn. Photo courtesy of Heidie Mitchell, Department of Physical Education, Kent State University.

method for teaching movement. The seed of what was to become the movement education program in the schools of the United States was being planted.

It is of interest to note, however, that since the 1920s such American leaders as Thomas Wood, Rosalind Cassidy, and Jesse Feiring Williams have been proposing concepts of physical education which now fall under the general rubric of movement education. In the 1930s a pioneer leader in dance, Margaret H'Doubler, proposed new concepts in dance and applied them to basic movement. These forward-looking educators were even then attempting to apply research findings in child growth and development and the behavioral sciences to physical education.[2]

Nevertheless, it was not until after World War II that international exchange programs and Anglo-American workshops in elementary school physical education served as the catalyst for the growing trend toward acceptance of movement education as a vastly different approach to the school program in physical education in this country. No doubt the effectiveness of the catalyst was increased by such factors as the apparent novelty of the approach to the education of the whole child; a growing dissatisfaction with elementary school physical education programs and their orientation toward sports and games, which left many youngsters woefully inadequate insofar as physical skill was concerned; and last, but far from least, the theories advanced by some psychologists and educators that motor learnings as the earliest learnings of the child, form the base from which all other learnings occur. Several kinds of therapy programs to aid youngsters with perceptual-motor defects (advocated by Kephart,[3] Doman,[4] Delacato,[5] and Frostig,[6] among others) have gained varying degrees of acceptance among educators and medical men.

THE PROGRAM TODAY

Although movement education as a curricular program is now hardly a new idea in the field of physical education, recurring questions among those in the profession indicate that confusion still exists about the purpose of the program, the definition of some of its specific terminology, and its place in the total spectrum of elementary school physical education.

If physical education is an academic discipline, then the conceptual approach to teaching is indicated. One of the most respected authorities

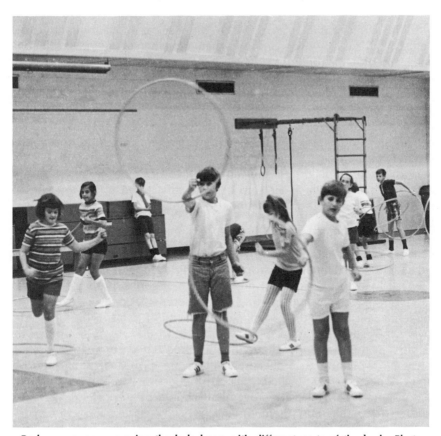

Body awareness — moving the hula hoop with different parts of the body. Photo courtesy of Lorie Coll and Ravenna (Ohio) City School System.

in the field of elementary school physical education in this country states: "Physical education, like every other discipline, can be organized so each child can gradually develop the main ideas of the discipline through the accumulation, comprehension, and synthesis of the related subject matter."[7] She then discusses three of the many concepts around which physical education can be organized.

1. Humans move to survive. This concept revolves around the "anatomical and physiological nature of man and his need to acquire physiological understanding and readiness for efficient movement."[8]

2. Humans move to discover and understand their environment. "As a child comes to understand his environment and use it successfully in movement, he acquires a more realistic body image and a more wholesome self-concept."[9]

3. Humans move to control and adjust to the environment. As children learn better to understand both themselves and the environment, they realize that the ability to "control and adjust" is based on efficient movement. "Thus he begins to work for the advantageous use of the elements of movement—space, time, force, and flow."[10]

With this conceptual approach, the purpose of movement education seems inextricably woven around what movement educators call *body management*—the ability of children to *control* their bodies in movement patterns because they *understand* the way the body can move in relation to the many forces exerted upon it. In other words, *movement sense,* the ability to move appropriately in a variety of situations, whether familiar or unfamiliar, is developed. Movement sense implies a feeling for movement based both upon kinetic experience and an informed observation of other children's movements.[11]

Movement education is the term used to describe the physical education curriculum which aims to achieve this purpose,[12] whereas *basic movement* refers to the foundational content of the program, a study of the elements of movement.

Movement exploration, the process by which children learn body management, is characterized by two main approaches, problem solving and guided discovery. The *problem-solving* approach is best described as an effort by the teacher to design an open-ended problem in such a manner that the youngster, through experimentation, discovers independently the best and most efficient movement pattern. In *guided discovery* the teacher plays a more direct role in that he or she poses the problem in such a manner that certain desired outcomes are likely.

In both of these approaches, teachers are more than interested observers. They actively teach throughout the lesson. Although they do not demonstrate how particular movements should be performed, they help children evaluate, help them understand why certain movements feel more comfortable or are efficient, and suggest possible changes.

The physical educator who is used to the traditional program in physical education at the elementary school level is often concerned about the refinement of skills necessary for specific sports, games, and dance. The movement education approach does not disregard such skill formation. (Refer again to Table 7.5.) Rather, the curriculum in movement education focuses on basic movement as the foundation on which fundamental skills are built. The transition from the fundamental skills to specific sports skills should then evolve not only more quickly but with a greater degree of perfection and understanding.

Not only the "traditionalist" in physical education but also the classroom teacher is often concerned about the paucity of structured game situations in a movement education program. Their concern is perhaps lessened when the movement educator explains that an analysis of most games reveals how space- and boundary-oriented they are, how many obstacles there are to overcome, how necessary it is to be aware of the directions in which one may move, how many different pathways can be taken to reach the goal, and how many different levels there are at which movement occurs. Understanding this, one can see that if children are well instructed in a good movement education program during their early experience with organized physical education, not only will they acquire the body management necessary for more effective refinement of sports skills at a later date, but they should also avoid some of the trauma and disappointment too often associated with the traditional method of teaching sports and games. Most of the rules and techniques in a typical sport such as basketball far exceed a child's ability to cope with them. Through movement education, with its emphasis on basic movement, a child should better learn to adjust to the constantly changing environment found in games. Success, a positive reinforcer, is thus more apt to be a result.[13]

The methodology of movement education is not restricted to the elementary school physical education program. In fact, a recent publication, *Sports Skills: A Conceptual Approach to Meaningful Movement*, describes how such methodology can be used in the teaching of skills specific to many different sports.[14] Although physical educators have for years been advocating the teaching of motor skills with an application of mechanical principles, few of them are well-versed in the guided discovery approach or in indirect methods of teaching. Therefore, their efforts have been mostly limited to teacher-directed goals. It seems clear, however, that more and more teachers at both the secondary and college level are experimenting with an approach to the teaching of sports and dance that encourages the learners to help set their own goals. Empirical data regarding the effectiveness of the problem-solving approach are becoming more available as college researchers attempt to discover and qualify the differences in results accruing from different teaching styles. For the most part, such studies tend to show the superiority of indirect methods of teaching over the traditional direct method. Selected studies are cited in references 15–19. The prospective teacher is urged to read carefully as many of them as possible. (All of the cited theses are available on microcards.) Russell's study is particularly interesting in that the results indicate that the "traditional" approach may even influence *skilled* performers negatively.

THE FUTURE OF MOVEMENT EDUCATION

There has been widespread dissatisfaction with the program of physical education in the schools today. The "movement movement" is undoubtedly one expression of this dissatisfaction as physical educators come to grips with poor programs, poor teaching, and poor attempts to conceptually organizing a body of knowledge revolving around human movement.

Whether the program of movement education, as described, is a passing fancy or an effective means toward the end of physically educated, self-directed, well-functioning human beings is, of course, still a matter of conjecture. It seems quite clear, however, that the program is gaining strength not only at the elementary school level but at upper educational levels as well. It also seems very clear that the ultimate worth of the program depends on the strength of the teachers in it. Unless the teachers truly understand the concepts underlying the discipline of physical education, they cannot master the exceptionally creative approach demanded and consequently cannot be effective in teaching. A very comprehensive recent treatment of both the content and the pedagogical implication of movement education, by Gilliom, should prove of inestimable help to the student or teacher who seeks to understand in greater depth this phase of the total physical education program.[20]

Evaluation of children in a movement education program, except subjectively and in relation only to themselves, is of little concern to the movement educator, who considers as one of the strengths of the program the fact that in the early phases of learning there is not single criterion of correct movement. Therefore the children experience only success. Of course, they can be guided to greater success by the teacher who understands how the child's body can most efficiently move within its own unique physical structure. However, evaluation of the *program* needs greater attention and a more sustained focus. Until movement educators can come up with more empirical evidence supporting some of their claims, it seems unlikely that universal acceptance will be forthcoming.

Locke[21,22] has written especially cogent critiques of movement education. His contention is that the future of movement education depends on (1) a more lucid delineation of why there continues to be dissatisfaction with the traditional program of physical education, (2) a definition of behavior-oriented objectives, (3) attention to teaching techniques, the strengths of which can be empirically demonstrated, and (4) the development of "well-publicized, attractive pilot programs" in the public schools that will catch the attention of school administrators, perhaps the only ones who can directly effect a change in the school curriculum.[23]

There seems to be little disagreement with the position that human movement must be the focus of the discipline.

> Since movement is used in some way, to some degree, in almost every task accomplished by human beings, the teaching of efficient movement becomes both an obligation and a challenge—a challenge to help each student develop the ability to use his body effectively in the performance of all tasks demanded of it, whether these tasks involve everyday living skills, work skills, or recreational skills.[24]

The proverbial writing on the wall has never been clearer. The very survival of the physical education program depends on the ability of the discipline to translate the writing into unified, defensible action.

STUDENT PROJECTS

1. Prepare an oral or written report on the studies cited in references 15–19.
2. Search out empirical studies dealing with the perceptual-motor therapy programs cited in references 3–6.
3. Review *Promising Practices in Elementary School Physical Education* by the American Alliance for Health, Physical Education and Recreation, and report on the scope of professional assistance and material available to the elementary school physical education teacher.
4. Visit an elementary school in which the movement approach is now used. Select any student to observe throughout the period. With a stopwatch keep track of the time that student is actually physically participating in the lesson. Repeat the procedure in an elementary school where physical education is taught "traditionally." Do the amounts of time differ significantly? Can you explain why?
5. Interview classroom teachers in the same elementary school. How do they compare the effectiveness of this type of curriculum with that of the "traditional" curriculum of games, and sports, as reflected by the youngsters' learning in physical education?
6. If possible, talk with some of the youngsters involved in a movement education curriculum to ascertain the depth and kinds of understandings of human movement they possess.

GLOSSARY OF TERMS

Movement education An approach to physical education which aims to help children achieve body management through an understanding of the elements of movement and the ways in which they affect their bodies in motion.

Body management   The ability of children to control their bodies as they move.

Elements of movement   Space, force, time, and flow.

   Space   The area in which movement occurs.

   Force   The effort required to move.

   Time   The speed with which movement occurs.

   Flow   The sequential connection of moving body parts.

Basic movement   The foundation structure of the movement program, with emphasis on gross motor skills, both locomotor and nonlocomotor.

Movement exploration   The process in movement education by which children learn body management.

Problem solving   A method of indirect teaching in which a problem is so designed that the child can discover independently, via experimentation, the most efficient movement pattern.

Guided discovery   A more teacher-directed approach by which an attempt is made to guarantee certain movement outcomes.

Conceptual approach   In methodology, an attempt to foster the child's comprehension of physical education through a synthesis of accumulated subject matter affective, cognitive, and psychomotor.

REFERENCES

1. W. McD. Cameron and Peggy Pleasance, *Education in Movement* (Oxford: Basil Blackwell, 1964), p. 4.

2. Elizabeth A. Ludwig, "Toward an Understanding of Basic Movement Education in the Elementary Schools," *JOHPER* **39** (March 1968), pp. 26–27.

3. D. H. Radler and Newell C. Kephart, *Success Through Play* (New York: Harper & Row, 1961).

4. Glenn Doman, *How to Teach Your Baby to Read* (New York: Random House, 1964.

5. Carl Delacato, *The Diagnosis and Treatment of Speech and Reading Problems* (Springfield, Ill.: Charles C Thomas, 1963).

6. Marianne Frostig and David Horn, *The Frostig Program for the Development of Visual Perception* (Chicago: Follett, 1964).

7. Naomi Allenbaugh, "Learning about Movement," *NEA Journal* **56** (March 1967), p. 48.

8. Ibid.

9. Ibid.

10. Ibid.

11. "The Concept of Physical Education," *British Journal of Physical Education* **1**:4 (July 1970), pp. 81–82. (Report of a Study Group).

12. Lorena Porter, *Movement Education for Children* (Washington: American Association of Elementary-Kindergarten-Nursery Educators, 1969), p. 5.

13. Heidie Mitchell, Unpublished lecture notes, Kent State University, 1970.

14. Beverly L. Seidel, Fay Biles, Grace Figley, and Bonnie Neuman, *Sports Skills: A Conceptual Approach to Meaningful Movement* (Dubuque, Iowa: W. C. Brown, 1975).

15. Iris L. Garland, "Effectiveness of Problem-Solving Method in Learning Swimming." Master's thesis, University of California, Los Angeles, 1960.

16. Gayle Gravelee, "A Comparison of the Effectiveness of Two Methods of Teaching a Four-Week Unit on Selected Motor Skills to First Grade Children." Master's thesis, University of North Carolina, Greensboro, 1965.

17. Marilyn R. Russell, "Effectiveness of Problem-Solving Methods in Learning a Gross Motor Skill." Master's thesis, University of Washington, 1967.

18. Martha Van Allen, "An Investigation Using the Movement Exploration Approach in the Teaching of Selected Swimming and Diving Skills." Doctoral diss., Springfield College, 1966.

19. Yvonne Zeigler, "A Comparison of Two Methods of Teaching Gymnastics." Master's thesis, University of Wisconsin, 1965.

20. Bonnie C. Gilliom, *Masic Movement Education for Children: Rationale and Teaching Units* (Reading, Mass.: Addison-Wesley, 1970).

21. Lawrence F. Locke, "Movement Education: A Description and Critique," in *New Perspectives of Man in Action* eds. R. C. Brown and B. J. Cratty (Englewood Cliffs, N.J.: Prentice-Hall, 1969), pp. 200–226.

22. Lawrence F. Locke, "The Movement Movement," *JOHPER* **37** (January 1966), pp. 26–27, 73.

23. Ibid., p. 73.

24. Marion R. Broer, *Efficiency of Human Movement* (Philadelphia: W. B. Saunders, 1966), p. 363.

SELECTED READINGS

Allenbaugh, Naomi. "Learning about Movement." *Journal of the National Education Association* **56** (March 1967), pp. 48–51.

American Association for Health, Physical Education and Recreation. *Promising Practices in Elementary School Physical Education.* Washington: National Education Association, 1969.

Ammons, R. B. et al. "Long Term Retention of Perceptual Motor Skills." *Journal of Experimental Psychology* **55** (April 1958), pp. 318–328.

Barrett, Kate Ross. *Exploration: A Method for Teaching Movement.* Madison, Wis.: College Printing and Typing, 1965.

Bilbrough, A., and Jones, P. *Physical Education in the Primary School.* London: University of London Press, 1963.

Bilodeau, Edward, and Bilodeau, Ina. "Motor-Skills Learning: Feedback." *Annual Review of Psychology* **12** (1961), pp. 243–259.

Broer, Marion R. *Efficiency of Human Movement.* Philadelphia: W. B. Saunders, 1966.

Broer, Marion R. "Movement Education: Wherein the Disagreement?" *Quest* **2** (April 1964), pp. 19–24.

Brown, Camille, and Cassidy, Rosalind. *Theory in Physical Education, A Guide to Program Change.* Philadelphia: Lea & Febiger, 1963.

Brown, Margaret C., and Sommer, Betty K. *Movement Education: Its Evolution and a Modern Approach.* Reading, Mass.: Addison-Wesley, 1969.

Cameron, W. McD., and Pleasance, Peggy. *Education in Movement.* Oxford: Basil Blackwell, 1964.

Carlquist, Maja. *Rhythmical Gymnastics.* London: Methuen, 1961.

Delacato, Carl. *Neurological Organization and Reading.* Springfield, Ill.: Charles C Thomas, 1966.

————. *The Diagnosis and Treatment of Speech and Reading Problems.* Springfield, Ill.: Charles C Thomas, 1963.

Doman, Glenn. *How to Teach Your Baby to Read.* New York: Random House, 1964.

Engels, Virgil. "Patterned Movements: A New Justification for Physical Education." *The Physical Educator* **25** (December 1968), pp. 170–172.

Espenschade, Anna S. "Perceptual-Motor Development in Children." *Academy Papers of the American Academy of Physical Education* **1** (March 1968), pp. 14–20.

Frostig, Marianne, and David Horn. *The Frostig Program for the Development of Visual Perception.* Chicago: Follett, 1964.

Garland, Iris L. "Effectiveness of Problem-Solving Method in Learning Swimming." Master's thesis, University of California, Los Angeles, 1960.

Gilliom, Bonnie C. *Basic Movement Education for Children: Rationale and Teaching Units.* Reading, Mass.: Addison-Wesley, 1970.

Gravelee, Gayle. "A Comparison of the Effectiveness of Two Methods of Teaching a Four-Week Unit in Selected Motor Skills to First Grade Children." Master's thesis, University of North Carolina, Greensboro, 1965.

Hanson, Margie. "Physical Education '73." *Instructor* **82** (January 1973), pp. 45–53.

Howard, Shirley, "Movement Education Approach to Teaching in English Elementary Schools." *Journal of Health, Physical Education and Recreation* **38** (January 1967), pp. 30–33.

Hunt, Valerie. "Movement Behavior: A Model for Action." *Quest* **2** (April 1964), pp. 69–91.

Knapp, B. *Skill in Sport.* London: Routledge and Kegan Paul, 1963.

Laban, Rudolf, and Lawrence, F. C. *Effort.* London: MacDonald and Evans, 1947.

Locke, Lawrence F. "Movement Education: A Description and Critique." In *New Perspectives of Man in Action,* edited by R. C. Brown and B. J. Cratty. Englewood Cliffs, N.J.: Prentice-Hall 1969, pp. 200–226.

————. "The Movement Movement." *Journal of Health, Physical Education and Recreation* **37** (January 1966), pp. 26–27, 73.

Lockhart, Aileene. "Prerequisites to Motor Learning." *Academy Papers of the American Academy of Physical Education* **1** (March 1968), pp. 1–13.

Ludwig, Elizabeth A. "Toward an Understanding of Basic Movement Education in the Elementary Schools." *Journal of Health, Physical Education and Recreation* **39** (March 1968), pp. 26–28, 77.

MacKenzie, Marlin M. *Toward a New Curriculum in Physical Education.* New York: McGraw-Hill, 1969.

Metheny, Eleanor. "How Does a Movement Mean?" *Quest* **8** (May 1967), pp. 1–6.

―――. "Only by Moving Their Bodies." *Quest* **2** (April 1964), pp. 47–51.

Mosston, Muska. *Developmental Movement.* Columbus, Ohio: Charles E. Merrill, 1965.

Piaget, Jean. *The Origins of Intelligence in Children.* New York: International Universities Press, 1966.

Porter, Lorena. *Movement Education for Children.* Washington: American Association of Elementary-Kindergarten-Nursery Educators, 1969.

Questions and Answers about Movement Education. ESEA—Title III Program of Movement Education for Plattsburgh (New York) Elementary Schools (Joan Tillotson, Project Director), 1968.

Radler, D. H., and Kephart, Newell C. *Success Through Play.* New York: Harper & Row, 1961.

Randall, Marjorie. *Basic Movement.* London: G. Bell, 1961.

Russell, Marilyn R. "Effectiveness of Problem-Solving Methods in Learning a Gross Motor Skill." Master's thesis, University of Washington, 1967.

Ryser, Otto. "Are We Guilty of Malpractice?" *Journal of Physical Education and Recreation* **47** (September 1976), 28–29.

Sage, George H. *Introduction to Motor Behavior,* Reading, Mass.: Addison-Wesley, 1971.

Seidel, Beverly L. et al. *Sports Skills: A Conceptual Approach to Meaningful Movement.* Dubuque, Iowa: W. C. Brown, 1975.

Siedentop, Daryl. *Physical Education: An Introductory Analysis.* Dubuque, Iowa: W. C. Brown, 1976.

Sturtevant, Mary. "Movement Efficiency and the Novice Swimmer." *The Physical Educator* **26** (March 1969), pp. 24–25.

Sweeney, Robert T. *Selected Readings in Movement Education.* Reading, Mass.: Addison-Wesley, 1970.

Van Allen, Martha. "An Investigation Using the Movement Exploration Approach in the Teaching of Selected Swimming and Diving Skills." Doctoral diss., Springfield College, 1966.

Zeigler, Yvonne. "A Comparison of Two Methods of Teaching Gymnastics." Doctoral diss., Springfield College, 1966.

Chapter 9
Current Trends
in Education

There is nothing permanent
except change.

HERACLITUS

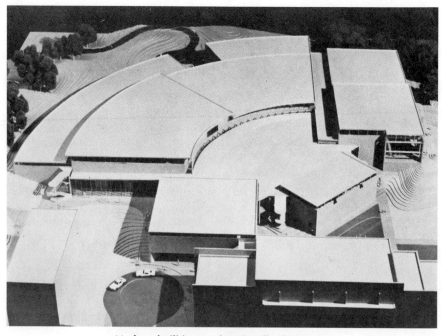

Modern facilities are functionally designed.
Photo courtesy of the School of Health, Physical Education and Recreation,
Kent State University.

THE SCHOOL program in physical education encompasses the largest single application of the discipline of physical education. Consequently, those who teach physical education need always to be aware of current philosophies of education as well as the latest trends based on such philosophy. Although it is not the purpose of this chapter to discuss educational philosophy per se, the changes which are taking place in education cannot be overlooked. In their commitment to change, many administrators are encouraging teachers to be innovative and creative, and they are fostering a climate conducive to experimentation. It is up to physical educators, then, to take advantage of such opportunities and prove once and for all that the dualism of mind and body is forever extinct, that their specialized field of learning can contribute to the objectives of all education, and that, indeed, their unique concerns are properly also concerns of all of education.

Some of the topics discussed cannot properly be called "current trends" since a few schools have employed them for many years. It seems safe to say, however, that the vast majority of schools either have not used them at all or else have incorrectly termed as such some modification of them. For example, one cannot truly identify a program as team-taught when the divider between boys' and girls' classes is removed and one teacher presents an activity while the other is responsible for discipline.

This chapter is devoted, then, to a discussion of selected current trends in education and of ways in which these new developments can be incorporated into the teaching of physical education. No attempt is made to place a value judgment on these innovations. Only after the theorists have fully explored what "ought" to be and the teachers have shown how such findings can be put into practice, can effective evaluation take place. For most of the trends discussed, that time has not yet arrived.

COEDUCATIONAL CLASSES

Some schools have offered coeducational classes in physical education, at least on occasion, for many years. Those schools which have not are now mandated by Title IX to do so. This fact seems to bother many physical education teachers and administrators, most often only because of a natural resistance to change. Given a real understanding of the theoretical foundation for such a program and time to work out some of the imperfections that inevitably accompany a break with tradition, it would seem that the advantages of scheduling classes on bases other than sex far outweigh the disadvantages.

Most of the disadvantages revolve around misconceptions (nourished by years of repetition and acceptance) such as the ideas that boys will

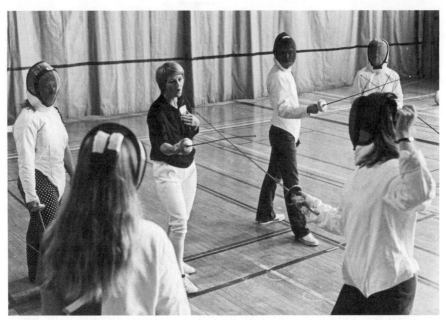

Coeducational classes are vital aspects of the total school program in physical education. Photo courtesy of Department of Physical Education, Kent State University.

not enjoy and/or learn in coeducational classes because girls are so inferior to them in skill; that girls will not accept a challenge to improve their skills because they are too embarrassed to perform in front of boys; that male teachers do not understand the female personality; that female teachers cannot handle disciplinary problems presented by boys; that female teachers prepare well for teaching responsibilities, whereas male teachers merely unlock the equipment and let the students play. All such misconceptions can be exposed as the myth they are in a properly conducted program under competent supervision.

The advantages of coeducational classes are legion. With the current emphasis on the "new physical education" and a program which features lifetime sports, it seems only reasonable to teach *students* instead of boys or girls. If the teaching-learning environment is always artificial— that is, separated by sex—how and when will boys and girls learn to participate together even as each sex learns to accept the *real* differences of the other? The teacher who had significant teaching strengths in specific activities ought to teach those activities to both sexes. Masculine and feminine stereotypes ought to disappear as boys learn that girls not only desire to excel but can hone their skills to a sufficiently high degree to defeat them on occasion. Such defeat ought not bruise the male ego; it has nothing whatsoever to do with maleness. If girls wish to be "members of the team," they ought to develop a better understanding of the male competitive spirit and, along with it, a more positive attitude about the development of skill and fitness. Male and female teachers ought to develop understanding and respect for each other and thus learn from each other so that all strive for the best possible instructional program. Only when such attributes as these, among others, are developed and nurtured can we expect students to learn about and adjust to "real life."

TEAM TEACHING

Team teaching is a concept that has arisen as one of the many possible answers in a search for creative and better methods of instruction in American schools. The concept has been variously defined but, in general, the following criteria must be met if the effort is to be considered team teaching.

1. A corps of two or more teachers (usually at least three and no more than eight).
2. Cooperative planning, instructing, and evaluating by the corps of teachers.
3. Involvement of one or more class groups (usually more than one).
4. Consideration given to special competencies of each member of the team.
5. Designation of a team leader.
6. Flexible arrangement of facilities, equipment, and time periods.

Actually, "team organization and planning" is a more appropriate title for this educational endeavor, since it is usual at any given moment for only one individual to be teaching. Misnamed or not, the concept seems to be gaining acceptance, so an exploration of some of its characteristics is warranted.

As indicated above, a team leader is usually designated. In such a situation, the corps is considered a "hierarchical team" with a definite chain of command from top to bottom, in contrast to a "cooperative team," all of whose members share equally in responsibilities.[1] Both types of organization have advantages, but most schools report less confusion when a team leader is appointed and job descriptions are formulated. Not all teachers wish to serve on a teaching team, nor are all teachers capable of performing well as part of a team. Therefore teachers must be chosen with care, and consideration should be given to such factors as willingness to accept peer and pupil criticism, dedication to self-improvement, ability to communicate well in large groups, in-depth knowledge and skill in the area involved, and ability to use instructional media and resources to their best advantage.

Paraprofessionals can play a large role in the concept of team teaching, and flexible scheduling is undoubtedly productive of the best learning. Both of these ideas are discussed separately later in this chapter.

It seems logical to assume that the cost of team teaching is somewhat higher than that of more traditional methods of instruction, although many of its proponents claim it is less expensive, *if properly conducted,* because large-group instruction takes care of more students at one time, less costly paraprofessionals are used to good advantage, individual study is fostered, and more efficient use of the facilities is made.

As is true with any instructional innovation, the attitude of the administration is probably the single most significant factor in the success or failure of a program. If the school principal, for example, not only is willing to try out new methods but actively encourages such experimentation on the part of the teachers, the program is likely to be successful. Obviously, such other factors as teacher interest and adequate preparation time are essential, but nothing else is so devastating as administrative apathy.

There is not an abundance of written material on team teaching in physical education; however, most authors of what material there is believe that its advantages are numerous. Among the more obvious ones are varying the teacher-pupil ratio according to the needs and abilities of the students, the competency of the teacher, and the available facilities; assigning the pupils according to their needs for a particular kind of instruction; fostering professional growth among the teachers, often with greater attendant camaraderie and unification; and motivating the student to more independent study of a better quality.

It is intriguing to reflect on the fact that many of the foregoing aspects of team teaching have been practiced for many years in one part of the total physical education program, varsity athletics. Football, for example, has often been called the best-taught subject in high school. In football, the team leader (head coach) calls together the rest of his corps of teachers (assistant coaches). They cooperatively plan their instruction program, taking into consideration the special competencies of the teachers (the defensive backfield coach, for example) and the needs and abilities of the students (defensive safety players who need considerable work on pass protection.) Then they set up a flexible arrangement of equipment and facilities to meet these special needs. For example, perhaps the safety men need to concentrate on pass protection, whereas the defensive ends need to practice rushing the quarterback. The entire teaching (coaching) team engages in cooperative evaluation of their product, and students (players) have the advantage as well as the responsibility for self-evaluation and self-improvement through the media of movies of their performance, execution charts kept by managers (paraprofessionals), instant replay television, and other means.

It is equally intriguing, as well as perplexing, to reflect on the fact that the same creative endeavors are not characteristic of the teaching in the required physical education program. The reasons are diverse, and discussion of them would require a great many pages. Perhaps the final answer lies in the fact that the typical physical educators have not "sold" their product—either to the school administration or to the public.

DIFFERENTIATED STAFFING

One of the most frequently voiced laments of teachers concerns being "freed to teach." The variety of nonteaching duties for which the typical teacher is responsible is so great that he or she often finds little time to prepare adequately for teaching. Then, too, there are extremely diverse teaching loads, often based on nothing more than an ill-conceived decision made a decade or two earlier. This problem is especially acute in physical education; the physical educator may have 1500 different student contacts a week, for example, whereas the mathematics teacher has "only" 600. Factors such as these underlie increasing teacher unrest and militancy.

Differentiated staffing, a concept which deals with the teacher as an individual but in an organizational context, is a "promising solution" to the problem of providing quality education by improving teacher efficiency.[2] It is predicated on the theory that the teacher is one of the most important elements in student learning and that it is at best a debilitating practice to treat all teachers alike, regardless of experience or talent, insofar as instructional responsibilities, advancement, and monetary rewards are concerned. Under a plan of differentiated staffing, teachers are treated according to their ability to perform specific tasks, and they are paid according to the complexity of those tasks. Teaching thus becomes a "career," and it is possible for a dedicated teacher to plan accordingly.

Basic to any plan of differentiated staffing is the involvement of teachers in decision-making processes and in the evaluation of their colleagues. It is perhaps fair to say that many teachers in the past have not wished to be involved in either of these ventures, particularly the latter, but the pattern is changing as better prepared, more brilliant teachers are actively involved in every part of the entire educational program.

Rand and English describe a differentiated-staffing model in which there are three basic areas of additional responsibility besides teaching: (1) "instructional management," in which a "senior teacher" functions as a learning engineer; (2) "curriculum construction," in which a "master teacher" is responsible for incorporating the latest research and educational theory into the curriculum; and (3) "staff teacher," who has advanced skill in applying research findings to the instructional act. In addition, there is an "associate teacher" category for the beginning teacher who needs to be brought along slowly under sympathetic, wise, and professional supervision.[3]

In a program of differentiated staffing, one can apply for a position at any of the three levels described above. The acquisition of such positions is based on qualifications for the specific responsibilities involved, and contractual arrangements differ in both length and remuneration. Advancement at any level is not automatic but is based on evaluation by colleagues. Merit pay, another trend in education, is perhaps basic to this plan.

The promises of differentiated staffing for all of education, including physical education, are many. The most significant may be the opportunity for increased professionalism and a higher degree of competence in that selected personnel are freed to develop certain responsibilities and functions for the good of all teaching personnel. The end result seems almost certain to be higher quality education for all through greater utilization of educational resources.

In physical education, one can visualize the department chairperson as the master teacher, the dedicated teacher with long experience at different educational levels as the senior teacher, the teacher with a minimum of a master's degree as a staff teacher, and the beginner as the associate teacher, who, if capable and interested, cannot help growing professionally under the protection and guidance of the others.

FLEXIBLE (MODULAR) SCHEDULING

Flexible scheduling is based primarily on two concepts: (1) students with differing needs and abilities should be scheduled in classes according to these differences; and (2) not all courses need the same amount of time, and the same courses may even need differing amounts of time on different occasions. For the implementation of such concepts, the school day is constructed around a specific period of time, called a module (or "mod"), which is perhaps fifteen to twenty minutes in length. The modules are then used as building blocks on which the master schedule is constructed. Whereas the traditional schedule cycles daily, the flexible schedule usually cycles weekly. Whereas the traditional schedule leaves little, if any, unscheduled time, the flexible schedule guarantees free time to the student to be used for individual study, whether preparing a "homework" assignment, practicing swimming skills, or conferring with teachers, who also have unscheduled time.

Four basic types of instructional groups are possible under flexible scheduling: large-group instruction, small-group instruction, independent study, and laboratory study. It is possible that most areas of instruction in physical education will use all four types in an integrated fashion. Let us say, for example, that all tenth graders, both boys and girls, meet together one day a week for two mods of large-group instruction. If their particular unit of study is tennis, they can hear lectures on the history, rules, etiquette, and training considerations for tennis, view films of tennis players in action, or hear lectures by guest tennis pros. On two other days of the week, boys and girls can meet separately or together in small groups for three or four mods of actual skill practice. On yet another day, an even smaller group that needs extra instruction because of basically poor motor skills can meet for one or two mods. In addition, the gymnasium and the tennis courts are open for indepen-

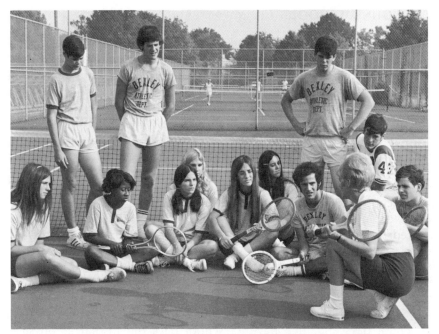

Tennis, an activity that lends itself well to coeducational instruction. Photo courtesy of the Ohio Association for Health, Physical Education and Recreation.

dent "study"—in this case, perhaps, practice on a backboard or on a rebound net.

It is fairly easy to see how team teaching and even differentiated staffing, as discussed earlier, fit into a flexible scheduling pattern. Not all teachers are equally competent to lecture to large groups, nor do all have the patience to work with low-skilled individuals. Not all teachers have enough free time to preview movies before they are shown or to research certain sociological factors surrounding the game of tennis.

Flexible scheduling, like other educational innovations, does away with many traditional aspects of schooling, the elimination of which some teachers find hard to accept. For example, there are no bells to signal the beginning and end of modules; students have a great deal more freedom, and they are responsible for its wise use; emphasis is placed on performance, and it matters little whether the student learned to "perform" in a large group or in independent study; and the scheduling of time, facilities, teachers, and students is too complex to be done manually.

There are, of course, disadvantages to flexible scheduling; however, if wisely used, this concept seems to be one that is truly productive of quality education through effective use of teaching talents, through greater responsibility of the students for their own education, through more rational use of time, and through complete utilization of facilities.

YEAR-ROUND SCHOOLS

The concept of year-round schooling, often called the extended school year, came into sharp focus around 1968 when soaring enrollments and overcrowded classrooms forced many schools to operate on double shifts or split sessions. Such operations are obviously detrimental to quality education, and concerned educationists, seeking an answer to the dilemma, turned to a concept which had been first tried in the 1800s. An extended school year is predicated upon the notion that it is wasteful to close schools for nearly half of each year (in most states children are required to attend school for 180 days); that it is less expensive to keep existing facilities open all year than to build new ones; that the traditional school calendar, based on the needs of an agrarian society, is now obsolete; and that educational enrichment opportunities can better be assured. Although today there is a more stable enrollment pattern, year-round schools are still popular and their proponents rationalize them based on improved educational opportunities for all boys and girls. In an extended school year, pupils attend three out of four quarters on a rotating basis. There are many variations of this plan, but perhaps the most popular is the so-called 45–15 plan where children are in attendance for 45 school days and then have 15 school days off. Insofar as physical education is concerned, such a plan seems meritorious on at least two counts: first, the shorter time in school is more conducive to offering a wider variety of lifetime sports; and second, many activities such as sailing and other aquatic sports can be offered because of the availability of additional facilities during the summer months.

MAINSTREAMING

One of the newer and more controversial practices in the public schools today is mainstreaming, integrating physically and mentally handicapped children into regular classes. Proponents of mainstreaming cite the following advantages: handicapped children learn to cope better with the real world if they are not isolated, they achieve more academically, and normal children learn better to understand the problems of the handicapped if they are exposed to them. Detractors say that regular teachers are not qualified to handle the special problems of the handicapped, class sizes become unmanageable, and the handicapped are ridiculed by their normal counterparts. Regardless of the pros and cons, mainstreaming is a growing practice and the physical educator can look forward to integrated classes. The wise student, it would seem, ought to become prepared for such teaching assignments.

THE USE OF PARAPROFESSIONALS

As mentioned earlier in this chapter, the typical teacher is faced with so many nonprofessional duties that he or she often has difficulty finding sufficient time to prepare adequately for instruction. Tax-conscious school patrons are beginning to realize that it is economically feasible to employ a number of paraprofessionals, sometimes called teaching aides, to perform nonteaching duties and thus free the higher-salaried professionals to do the jobs for which they are most qualified.

A paraprofessional in education can be defined as a mature adult who is trained to perform various nonteaching tasks in an educational institution. The persons who may qualify are quite varied: homemakers who want only part-time jobs, college students who are helping to finance their education, retired persons who are interested in "keeping in touch" with youth and their education, and others. The tasks they can be trained to perform include typing, filing, recording test scores, issuing locks and lockers, taking attendance, supervising playground and recess activities, caring for and repairing equipment, constructing bulletin boards, showing audiovisual aids, and *assisting* in instruction.

Two criteria in the definition of a paraprofessional cannot be emphasized too strongly. First, a "mature adult" is a necessity because of legal liability ramifications. For example, if a paraprofessional is supervising some safety aspect of individual practice of a physical education skill, he or she must be "reasonably prudent," according to law, since he or she is operating "in loco parentis." Second, being "trained to perform" is a prerequisite to effective performance. Some nonteaching duties, such as locker and shower room supervision, may seem too simple to require training, but problems, some of them quite personal in nature, arise on occasion, and the paraprofessional who is trained to recognize them and to deal professionally with them can contribute to overall quality education.

The advantages of using paraprofessionals are many and obvious. Perhaps the biggest disadvantage is that, unless caution is exercised, the teacher is apt to limit severely his or her personal exposure to students. No dedicated teacher will allow this to happen, however.

NEW CONCEPTS IN FACILITIES FOR PHYSICAL EDUCATION

Modular construction. Modular or "systems" construction consists of bringing together a number of prefabricated subsystems, sometimes called "pods," which make it possible to erect a school building in a matter of a few months and at a considerable reduction in cost. Reduced cost alone is perhaps sufficient justification for such construction, but one of the greatest advantages is its extreme flexibility. Interior space can be readily rearranged by moving partitions and relocating lighting, ventilation and heating ducts, and other components. Such renovation is in no way as costly as is the remodeling of conventional school buildings.[4]

Dome-shaped and air-supported structures. The number of structures of this type is increasing each year. A dome-shaped building is compara-

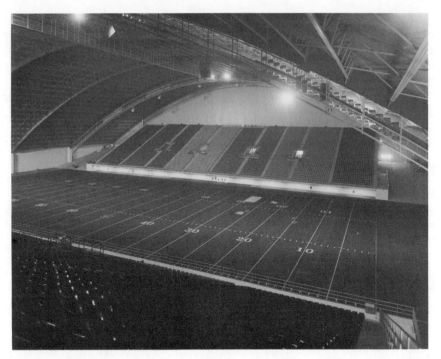

Interior of Idaho State University Minidome, a new concept in an all-weather, low-cost sports facility. Photo courtesy of Department of Physical Education, Idaho State University.

tively less expensive than a traditional one to erect, and it is usually more readily adaptable for multiple use. Spectator facilities must not usurp instructional space. With good planning, a structure that accommodates both can be erected. As for air-supported structures, researchers are working on a system to reinforce an "air only" structure by the use of cable systems which transmit forces to the ground rather than to the enclosure itself and which use inexpensive plastic sheets as membranes rather than coated fabric.[5]

Artificial surfaces. Artificial surfaces have now been developed for almost all types of physical education instruction. The various synthetic grass surfaces were the first on the market, and many football fields are now covered with such turf. Although there is not universal agreement on the value of artificial turf, its use to date has fairly well established the fact that it takes a maximum of hard and diverse wear with a minimum of maintenance.

In addition to artificial surfaces on playing fields, new surfaces are beginning to replace traditional wooden floors in gymnasia as well as dirt areas in fieldhouses. There are many different types of surfaces, but basically they are all constructed from some type of plastic. According to the various manufacturers, some of the advantages of these surfaces

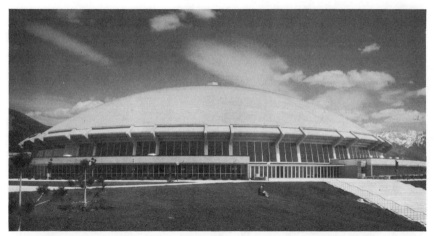

University of Utah sports and special events center, seating capacity 15,000. Photo courtesy of Department of Physical Education, University of Utah.

are: (1) they are more durable than wood, and they require less maintenance; (2) all types of balls bounce true with no dead spots; (3) cleats and spikes cannot harm the surface, although they are unnecessary because of its nonslip nature; and (4) there is a sharp reduction in fatigue and in the danger of injury.

Ice arenas. Facilities for ice skating are becoming ever more popular, and they can be incorporated into an all-purpose building, as discussed above. The newest innovation, perhaps the most adaptable and yet the least expensive, is plastic ice. Experiments are now being conducted, and many traveling ice show companies use plastic ice when true ice is unavailable.

Greater flexibility combined with lower costs is of extreme importance in physical education. Facilities for physical education are specialized and extremely expensive; therefore the best construction plan is on that allows for maximum use at minimum cost. Some of the proposed innovations in gymnasium construction include motorized rolling bleachers that serve as movable walls, huge overhead doors on outside walls so that in good weather they can be raised to include the outdoor area in the instructional space, and pivot walls that can serve as storage areas, bulletin boards, projection screens, etc., as well as wall space for such games as handball.[6]

INSTRUCTIONAL MEDIA

It would be remiss in a chapter on current trends not to include discussion of the various educational or instructional media that are prevalent today. The knowledge explosion is but one factor that has fostered the establishment of an instructional media center to replace more traditional

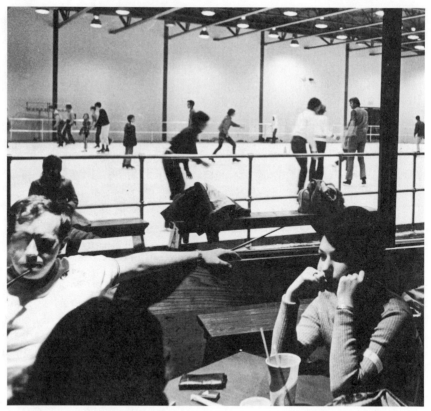
Facilities for ice skating provide worthwhile leisure time opportunities. Photo courtesy of Kent State University News Service.

audiovisual centers. The increase in the types, numbers, and sophistication of learning aids is also significant. This factor alone dictates central administration of all instructional materials and services for optimum and efficient use. In many schools, the instructional media center is a vital adjunct of the library.

The functions of such a center include the circulation of various kinds of materials, printed and otherwise; production of materials which teachers request, such as slides and filmstrips; and in-service education not only to acquaint teachers with what is available but also to instruct them in the preparation and use of their own materials. In physical education, for example, instant replay television has potential use that is still largely untapped. A very important premise on which effective centers operate is that all resources are readily available to students as well as to teachers. This concept demands space in the center itself where individuals can use the various media available.

Instructional media centers are vital at every level of education, kindergarten through college. Such centers, as well as the media contained within them, naturally become more complex at higher educational levels.

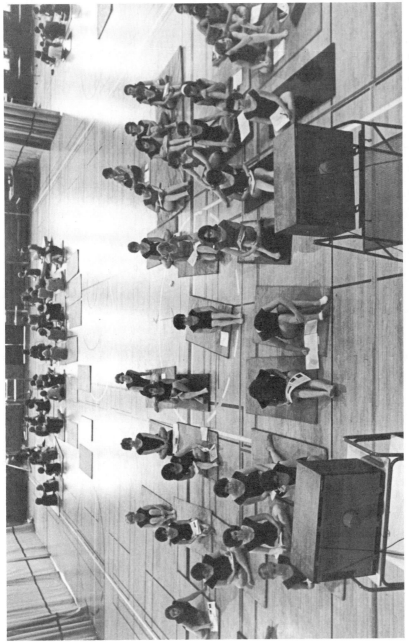

Television as an aid to instruction. Photo courtesy of Department of Physical Education, Kent State University.

It is also obvious that highly competent, trained individuals are needed if the centers are to function properly. Many universities now offer majors or at least minors in instructional media which lead to certification in the area. The demand for teachers educated to design and operate instructional media centers can only increase as many of the other current trends discussed in this chapter become accepted as vital to effective education.

SUMMARY

It is unfortunately true that programs in physical education seem often not to keep pace with changing patterns in education. Why this situation exists is debatable. The reason may be that the school administrator does not conceive of physical education and other "special" subjects as important enough to be considered in overall school change. Or perhaps the physical educator is not creative enough to realize how innovations can be applied effectively in his or her program. The fact remains that the school program in physical education is *education,* and therefore, even though it has concerns uniquely its own, it must also be cognizant of current educational philosophy and of the innovations which characterize such philosophy. Virtually all philosophers of education today subscribe to a theory of educating the whole child, and they contend that such education is a process of using all one's faculties cognitively, affectively, and psycho-motorially.

There is nothing inherently magic in change, nor should proposed innovations be adopted merely to be fashionable. Nevertheless, it is undeniably true that American schools can stand much improvement, and if some of the current trends seem productive of good, they should be tried and thoroughly evaluated, and on the basis of that evaluation, they should be maintained, altered, or discarded. We cannot overlook the fact that in any commitment to change, the responsibility for proving that one's special educational field is truly educational lies on the shoulders of each individual teacher. And teacher-coaches of physical education have many things going for them that should aid in the educative process. Not the least of them is a shared social involvement between teacher and student in the study of human movement that, if well nurtured, should foster genuine learning.

STUDENT PROJECTS

1. List the advantages and disadvantages of modular scheduling for physical education. If possible, visit a school with each type of scheduling: modular and "traditional." Report on conversation with both students and teachers regarding their evaluation of the type of scheduling they use.

2. If the visits suggested above are impossible, elicit reactions from class members who attended high schools with both types of scheduling.
3. List the advantages and disadvantages of team teaching in physical education. What reasons are given in the literature for the fact that many physical educators seem to shy away from this type of teaching?
4. Visit the instructional media center at your university. Report to the class on the types of services available and the ways in which such services might be implemented at the high school or elementary school level.
5. Survey a sampling of physical education teachers, athletic coaches, and intramural directors in your area to get their reactions to the advantages and disadvantages of artificial surfaces.
6. Start a collection of physical education facility plans including pictures and architects' drawings.
7. List the advantages and disadvantages of mainstreaming in physical education for the student, the teacher.

GLOSSARY OF TERMS

Team teaching   A program in which two or more teachers cooperatively plan, instruct, and evaluate a class or combination of classes.

Paraprofessionals   Mature individuals with training in nonprofessional tasks who are employed to assist the professional in a particular field.

Differentiated staffing   A plan whereby staff members are assigned different levels of responsibility, including teaching, according to their specific abilities.

Modular or flexible scheduling ("mods")   Arrangement of the school day into segments of time (modules) which can be combined differently according to the needs of the subject and/or the student.

Modular or systems construction ("pods")   The use of prefabricated or precut units in erecting school facilities.

Instructional media center   A center where various kinds of teaching and learning aids are housed. These aids range from traditional materials, such as films and slides, to models, printed materials, and instant replay television apparatus.

Mainstreaming   The integration of physically and mentally handicapped children into regular classes.

REFERENCES

1. Judson T. Shaplin and Henry F. Olds, eds. *Team Teaching* (New York: Harper & Row, 1964), p. 116.

2. Fenwick English, *Et Tu, Educator, Differentiated Staffing?* (Washington: National Commission on Teacher Education and Professional Standards, National Education Association, 1969), pp. 1–5.

3. John M. Rand and Fenwick English, "Towards a Differentiated Teaching Staff," *Phi Delta Kappan* **49** (January 1968), pp. 264–269.

4. Velma Adams, "The Trend to School Building Systems," *School Management* (August 1969), p. 30.

5. P. R. Theibert, "New Ideas in Physical Education Facilities," *Physical Education Supplement* (Croft Educational Services, 1970), p. 4.

6. Lamar Kelsey, Fred Kolflat, and Robert Schaefer, "New Generation Gyms," *Nation's Schools* **84** (December 1969).

SELECTED READINGS

Adams, Velma. "The Trend to School Building Systems." *School Management* (August 1969), pp. 24–30, 49–54.

———. "Why Systems Can't Miss." *School Management* (September 1969), pp. 66–73.

Barbee, Don. *Differentiated Staffing: Expectations and Pitfalls.* Washington: National Commission on Teacher Education and Professional Standards, National Education Association, 1969.

Christensen, D. Louis. "How 'Mod' Can You Get?" *Ideas Educational* **6** (Winter 1968), pp. 9–14.

Dennard, Rebecca. "The 12-Month School Year: An Opportunity for Health and Physical Education Programs." *Bulletin, NASSP,* (April 1975).

Elliott, Patricia. "The Beneficial Outcomes of Requiring Coeducational Programs." *Journal of Health, Physical Education and Recreation* **43** (February, 1972), p. 35.

English, Fenwick. *Et Tu, Educator, Differentiated Staffing?* Washington: National Commission on Teacher Education and Professional Standards, National Education Association, 1969.

Fenwick, James. "The Extended School Year: Questions to Think About." *The Education Digest* **XLI** (September 1975).

"Focus on Facilities." *Journal of Physical Education and Recreation* **47**:7(September 1976).

Georgiades, William. "Team Teaching: A New Star, Not a Meteor." *Journal of the National Education Association* **56** (April 1967), pp. 14–15.

Gickling, E. E., and Theobald, John. "Mainstreaming: Affect or Effect?" *Journal of Special Education* **9** (Fall 1975).

Kelsey, Lamar; Kolflat, Fred; and Schaefer, Robert. "New Generation Gyms." *Nation's Schools* **84** (December 1969), 15 pp. [unnumbered].

Mager, Robert F. *Preparing Instructional Objectives.* Palo Alto, Calif: Fearon, 1962.

Martin, Edwin W. "Some Thoughts on Mainstreaming." *Exceptional Children* **41** (November 1974).

Pearson, Neville P., and Butler, Lucius, eds. *Instructional Materials Centers.* Minneapolis: Burgess, 1969.

Pie, Harry E. "What Flexible Scheduling Is All About." *Journal of Health, Physical Education and Recreation* (March 1967), p. 30.

Rand, John M., and English, Fenwick. "Toward a Differentiated Teaching Staff." *Phi Delta Kappan* **49** (January 1968), pp. 264–268.

Reams, David, and Bleier, T. J. "Developing Team Teaching for Ability Grouping." *Journal of Health, Physical Education and Recreation* **39** (September 1968).

Resick, Matthew C., Seidel, Beverly L.; and Mason, James. *Modern Administrative Practices in Physical Education and Athletics.* Reading, Mass.: Addison-Wesley, 1970.

Ridine, Leonard M. "The Paraprofessional in Physical Education." *The Physical Educator* (October 1970), pp. 114–117.

Sadowski, Gregory M. "Flexible Modular Scheduling Allows for Student Choice of Independent Study Units." *Journal of Health, Physical Education and Recreation* **42** (September 1971), p. 25.

Shaplin, Judson T., and Olds, Henry F., eds. *Team Teaching.* New York: Harper & Row, 1964.

Sullivan, Alice, and Savastano, Orlando L. "Teacher Aides in Physical Education." *Journal of Health, Physical Education and Recreation* (May 1969), pp. 26–28.

Theibert, P. R. "New Ideas in Physical Education Facilities." *Physical Education Supplement.* Croft Educational Services, 1970.

Trump, J. Lloyd. "Changing School to Serve Individuals Better in HPER." Multilithed. Washington: National Association of Secondary School Principals, 1970.

————. "Evaluating Pupil Progress in Team Teaching." Multilithed. Washington: National Association of Secondary School Principals, 1970.

————. "How Excellent Are Teaching and Learning in your School?" Multilithed. Washington: National Association of Secondary School Principals, 1970.

————. "Presentations and Other Types of Large-Group Instruction." Multilithed. Washington: National Association of Secondary School Principals, 1970.

Von Bergen, Enid. "Flexible Scheduling for Physical Education." *Journal of Health, Physical Education and Recreation* (March 1967), p. 31.

Wiley, W. Deane, and Bishop, Lloyd K. *The Flexibly Scheduled High School.* West Nyack, N.Y.: Parker, 1968.

Chapter 10
Athletics
in School
and Society

Participation in sound athletic programs, we believe,
contributes to health and
happiness, physical skill and
emotional maturity, social
competence and moral
values.

EDUCATIONAL POLICIES
COMMISSION, NATIONAL
EDUCATION ASSOCIATION

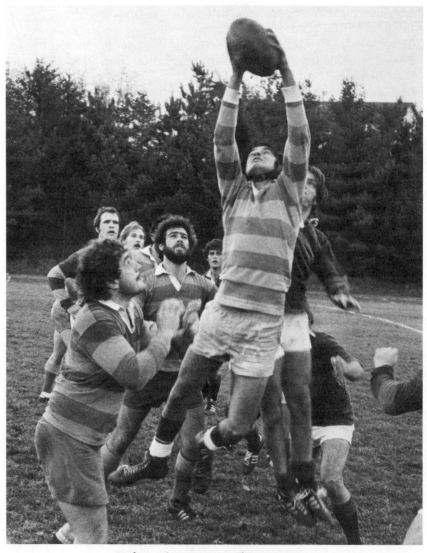

Rugby, a vigorous sport. Photo courtesy
of Kent State University Rugby Club.

T HE PLACE of athletics in so-
ciety, but more particularly in the schools, is an issue which has been
debated for many years. Arguments from its proponents at one end of
the value continuum espouse for athletics the same objectives as for all
of education. Its detractors at the other end of the continuum insist that
athletics is merely one aspect of show business and, as such, should be
divorced from the American educational enterprise. No doubt each of
these viewpoints has some merit. A program of athletics properly conducted has invaluable and almost limitless opportunities for meeting
many of the objectives which education deems desirable. On the other
hand, the same program improperly conducted can in no way be evaluated as educational, and therefore the "show business" connotation is
probably appropriate. Why is there such a divergence of viewpoints
about the school program of athletics? Perhaps the best way to answer
this question is to trace briefly the development of organized athletics;
to discuss the present school program, its values and its problems; and,
finally, to digest current trends and assess the future. Although the treatment is school-oriented, the role of athletics in society has an influence
on the school program and vice versa.

HISTORY OF ORGANIZED ATHLETICS

The early settlers brought some sports and games with them to the New
World, but there was very little in the way of organized athletics in the
communities and none in the schools until after the first quarter of the
nineteenth century.

There is less than complete agreement on the specific origins of many
sports and games, but the following statements regarding three of America's better-known sports activities are generally accepted.

Baseball, America's so-called national game, evolved from cricket and
rounders, and both Doubleday and Cartwright are given some credit for
its invention or development. The first organized team was the Knicker-
bocker Baseball Club of New York, founded in 1845. The first college
game was played between Amherst and Williams in 1859.

The present game of American football developed directly from
soccer and indirectly from rugby. Although the National Collegiate Athletic Association (NCAA) celebrated the hundredth anniversary of football
in 1969, in all probability, the 1869 game between Rutgers and Princeton
was a soccer game.

The invention of basketball by Naismith in 1891 filled a need for a
game that could be played indoors during the long winter months, when
football, soccer, and baseball could not be played.

While these and other sports were developing, the European programs of physical education were being introduced into American schools.

Sports activities were conducted in the schools by the citizens of the community and by unsupervised high school and university students. School played school, town played town, and many a playing field at times took on the look of a battleground. Football evolved into an especially rough sport, and the games became so dangerous that they were abolished for years by the faculties of Harvard and Yale. This roughness had reached a climax by the year 1905, when President Theodore Roosevelt called a meeting of representatives from Yale, Princeton, and Harvard to discuss the future of the game. That action can be considered the first real attempt to control athletic programs.

Beginnings of Athletic Controls

In spite of the difficulties encountered, athletics developed rapidly and by 1879 had reached such proportions that there arose a need for some kind of control. A direct result was the formation of the National Association of Amateur Athletes of America, an organization which developed into the Amateur Athletic Union (AAU) in 1888.

In 1905 the Chancellor of New York University, Henry McCracken, called a meeting of the nation's colleges to decide the fate of college football. Twenty-eight colleges were represented, and the groundwork was laid for the formation of the present National Collegiate Athletic Association (NCAA), founded in 1910. The most important agreement reached was that the conduct of athletics was to be left to the discretion of duly authorized school authorities, but such aspects as recruiting, subsidization, schedules, and tournaments were to be controlled.

In order to effect such control, most schools formed athletic boards of control or athletic councils. This type of administrative arrangement still operates on many college campuses and in many secondary schools. In the years that followed the formation of the AAU and the NCAA, interest not only in participating in but also in watching sports was highly evident among students and citizens of the communities. The affluence that followed World War I increased this interest. A Carnegie Foundation report entitled *American College Athletics,* issued in 1929, disclosed a shocking turn toward professionalism in all aspects of college sports.[1] The disclosure of scandals in recruiting athletes and subsidizing them by means of scholarships threatened the very existence of athletics in the school program. Athletic conferences were forced into a policing action in order to survive. Shortly after this report was issued, however, the United States suffered through the "Great Depression," and the drastic changes in the economy that followed served to remove the pressure of th critical issues facing competitive athletics. There have been minor athletic scandals since that period but perhaps nothing to match the disclosures in 1929.

NCAA-AAU-AIAW Conflicts

In recent years both the NCAA and the AAU have developed into power-ful organizations for the control of amateur athletics. The NCAA was formed to promote college and university athletic programs, whereas the AAU deals with amateur athletic programs outside educational insti-tutions. Under the circumstances, there seems to be little ground for dissent, but problems do arise in the selection of teams and coaches to take part in international competition, including the Olympics. The AAU has the official approval of the International Olympic Committee to select team members, team coaches, meet sites, and times. However, the training ground for many of the activities is the college and university athletic program. Furthermore, many of the athletes competing for team membership are attending colleges and universities on athletic grants-in-aid, and at times the NCAA and the AAU codes are in conflict. And with burgeoning athletic opportunities for females yet another organiza-tion, the Association of Intercollegiate Athletics for Women (AIAW), is challenging the NCAA for control of competitive programs for women at the college level. A joint committee representing both groups has been appointed to study the problem. Unfortunately, in all such conflicts, it is the student athlete who suffers. The problems are not insurmountable, but they are significant enough to have fostered governmental interven-tion at the federal level. One must hope, for the good of organized sport, both at home and abroad, that reasonable people will come together and resolve their conflicts.

EDUCATIONAL VALUES OF INTERSCHOOL ATHLETICS

The instructional program in physical education is an integral part of the curricular offerings of any school. And the field of physical education can point with pride to the fact that it was one of the first areas to extend its offerings into cocurricular activities, such as intramurals, extramurals, and varsity sports. All of these programs can lay claim to meeting par-ticular and individualized needs of students.

The intramural program, largely sports-oriented, is conducted "within the walls" of a particular educational institution. Its participants are usually semiskilled individuals, interested in engaging to a greater extent in some of the activities learned in the physical education class. Hence intramurals are often referred to as the physical education laboratory.

Extramural participation extends beyond a specific school, but usually competition in this category is informally organized and conducted. An example of extramural competition is a sports day in which two or more schools compete against each other in one or more activities. The teams from the schools are not of varsity caliber, but they may be the intra-mural winners in a particular sport in their respective schools.

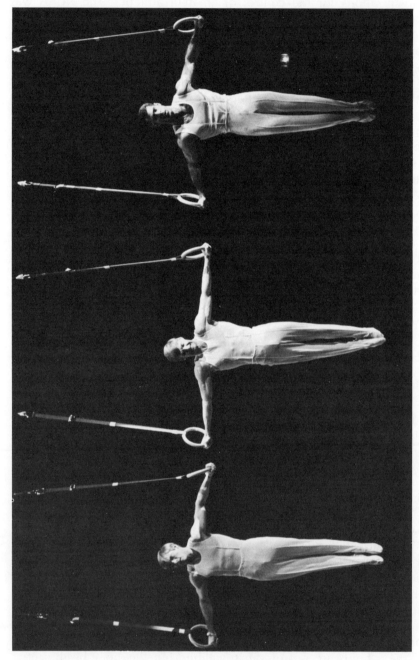

Gymnasts display the skill necessary for varsity competition. Photo courtesy of Kent State University Gymnastics Team.

The varsity team is a highly select group, representing a superior skill level, which receives extra coaching for the purpose of engaging in an interschool program of competitive athletics. It is in the varsity athletics that the exceptional students have the opportunity to develop their talent further and to measure themselves against other similarly gifted individuals. The varsity athlete is somewhat like the student who develops his or her speaking ability and enters forensic contests, the student musician who is a member of the concert band, and the student thespian who stars in school dramatic productions.

Many values are possible outcomes of such programs, but none can be guaranteed, of course. If the leadership is sound and if the program is kept within a justifiable educational perspective, the following values —in addition to the obvious ones revolving around physical fitness and a healthy body skilled in movement—seem to be possible outcomes from participation in athletics.

1. *Moral and social values.* It is possible to learn fair play, courage, justice, democratic skills, etc., in an atmosphere where social class, religion, color, and creed pale into insignificance as *human* values shine brightly through. Competition, conflict, and cooperation are all inherent in our society. In a wisely conducted program of interschool athletics, competitive and cooperative behavior can be maximized while conflict is at the same time being minimized.

2. *Intellectual values.* The opportunities to think critically and constructively are unparalleled in competitive athletics, in which there is constant need to make decisions with physical, social, and moral ramifications.

3. *Emotional values.* In a society in which pressures and tensions are so great that emotional illness is a national problem, it is helpful to be able to learn to adjust to pressure in a game situation. In addition, self-perception of one's body image—in other words, feeling at home in one's own body—is necessary for psychological well-being.

4. *Cultural values.* Using the body as a means of creative self-expression is today recognized to be just as "cultural" as expressing oneself through such other media as art, music, and drama.

5. *Vocational values.* A program of interschool athletics can serve as a vocational laboratory for future physical educators, coaches, and professional athletes. In addition, many of the attributes learned in such a program are important to later success in other vocational pursuits.

Thus most, if not all, of the objectives inherent in education are obtainable in a well-rounded, diversified curricular and cocurricular program of physical education. However, the interschool program in competitive athletics, theoretically the culmination of a sound instructional program in physical education, seems often to have received undue emphasis—to such an extent that the entire program, including interschool competition, is in danger of collapse. No area of study deserves the title "educational" if it uses most of its resources, human and other-

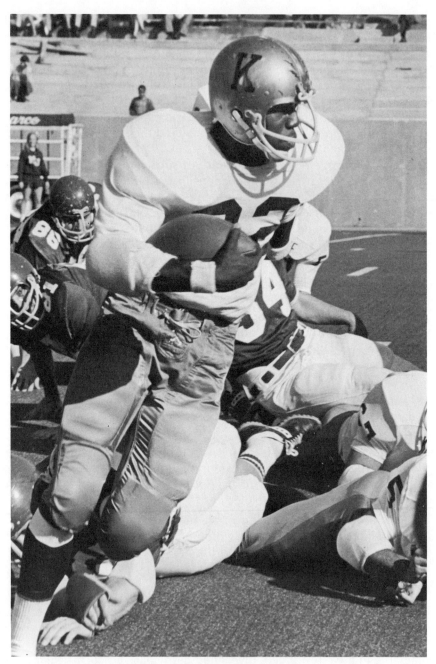

Football combines individual effort with teamwork. Photo courtesy of Kent State University Department of Intercollegiate Athletics.

wise, to serve the talented minority. What, then, are some of the problem areas in interschool athletic programs, and what can be done to eliminate them?

THE PROBLEMS IN ATHLETICS

Because athletics are an integral part of the community and a rallying point for both school and community spirit, the values in athletics too often become distorted. The distortion may begin in the school with coaches who sometimes *use* athletes as stepping-stones to further their own coaching careers. It is helped along by the school's administrative echelon, which makes one set of rules for athletes and another set for the remainder of the student body. The distortion is further nurtured by the community, which demands victory over the neighboring community —even to the point of insisting that a coach be fired if the wins do not greatly exceed the losses. And finally, the pressure comes from those parents who enjoy the vicarious thrill of athletic success by sharing the glory of victory with sons and daughters who are team members.

Another problem arises from the fact that the interschool athletic program, as an extra or cocurricular activity, must be largely if not entirely self-sustaining financially. Thus it is mandatory to have good gate receipts, and seemingly, this result can be accomplished only by fielding winning teams. In order to ensure that goal, action is taken which brings about many of the abuses of the program: lax eligibility standards, improper recruiting, illegal subsidizing, and other unethical coaching practices.

Yet another nagging question relative to keeping the program in an education perspective revolves around the age and grade level at which interschool sports should be initiated. Although selfish perpetuators of the feeder system would begin the process in kindergarten, there is no supportive evidence to indicate either that a need exists for interscholastic athletic programs at the elementary school level or that such early participation produces superior athletes at a later date. Nevertheless, the arguments that outside agencies sponsor it (for example, Little League baseball and Peewee football) seems sufficient to sway the administration in some school systems. Overlooked is the fact that such programs are adult-inspired, adult-motivated, and adult-controlled. Such programs do not permit children to enjoy the discovery and thrill of play in an unstructured atmosphere, and at the same time they severely limit participation. A strong intramural program permits the participation and development of all who wish to compete. In the long run, this practice is productive of a better interschool program.

The program of interscholastic athletics at the junior high school level is so entrenched that it is now almost unquestionably accepted in spite of research evidence which militates against *unrestricted* programs, especially in the contact sports. Much research is still needed concerning injuries to the bones during periods of growth and concerning the possibil-

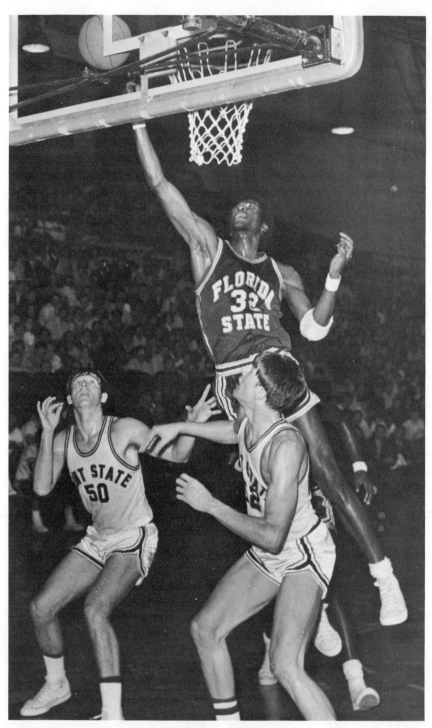

Basketball, a game for the well-conditioned athlete. Photo courtesy of Kent State University Department of Intercollegiate Athletics.

ities that interference with normal growth patterns can be traced to competitive athletics. Just as important is the unanswered question of the result of the emotional impact on young students due to tensions in competitive situations. Since it is unlikely that these programs will cease, it is mandatory that properly educated teacher-coaches be placed in positions of responsibility for their organization and administration.

Perhaps the biggest problem in interscholastic athletics at the senior high school level is that the program is so firmly entrenched in the minds and hearts of the citizens of the community that it is difficult for them to consider sports as education or as recreation. Instead they view the program as entertainment, and since they have such a vested interest in it and its participants, they tend to compare it to professional programs or at least to successful college programs. The National Federation of State High School Athletic Associations decries such attitudes and its members profess a belief that the high school athletic program must be confined within an educational framework. The Federation's beliefs are identified by its Executive Secretary as follows:

First, we believe that the nature of a nation's sports program reflects, to a large degree, the nation's physical well-being and its physical interests. . . .

Second, we believe in competition. It is beneficial for the highly skilled to compete, for the less skilled to compete, for the moderately skilled to compete. A desire to win is good, and most benefits occur when extreme effort is made; casual effort does not result in desirable benefits! We believe that there is a difference between recreational sports and competitive sports. And we believe further that competition should be regulated by standards.

Third, we believe that we should win according to the rules and that ethical practices should not be abused or voided in order to win. A program that is properly administered, even though it is competitive, will give the educational benefits we are striving for.

Fourth, we believe that a program with both breadth and depth is needed. There should be a great many sports opportunities for high school students and students should have a choice of the activity in which they want to participate. We believe that there is need for many teams on various levels. Not all students want to participate in programs that are highly competitive. Some students do not care about this kind of activity; some are not interested in making the sacrifices that are necessary if they are to excel.

Fifth, we believe that sportsmanship is taught and that the objectives we hope to attain can be reached only when sportsmanship is given a consideration. We believe that current approaches to sportsmanship are often "namby-pamby." Even with the fear of oversimplifying this important area, we suggest that there are three standards for sportsmanship. You can have acceptable sportsmanship generally if you will play the game according to the rules, both the spirit of the rules and the actual rules. If you win you do not gloat over it. If you lose you do not alibi. We believe that some "window dressing" is insincere in the sportsmanship area, that it is unnecessary. Furthermore, it contributes to a weakness or a fault of our competitive program. We think that it is artificial and we believe that sportsmanship is dependent upon sincerity.

Finally, we believe that personal and social values can be attained in sports competition but that these objectives are not automatic and, to a great degree, they depend upon leadership.[2]

In order to meet desirable standards of interscholastic programs at secondary school levels, it seems that *minimally* a coach's background should reflect a study of the growth and developmental patterns of students and the medical aspects of sports, as well as a basic knowledge of the sport he or she is coaching. In its concern for the student athlete, the State of Ohio Board of Education, in September 1970, passed the following resolution.[3]

RESOLUTION "A"

WHEREAS, this Board has adopted A Guide for the Development of a School Activity Program, and

WHEREAS, said Guide provides in part that:
Student participation in interscholastic athletics is restricted to those enrolled in the seventh grade or above. Students in grades seven and eight should not be permitted to participate in interscholastic athletics except when a broad and comprehensive program in physical education and intramurals exists for all boys and girls. The number of contests and types of sports, in which individual students participate, shall be kept at a minimum. Every control needed to insure the health, safety and physical well-being of the participant in interscholastic athletics shall be provided.

and

WHEREAS, the health and safety of students participating in interscholastic athletics continues to be a vital concern of this Board,

NOW THEREFORE BE IT RESOLVED that the following addition be made to said Guide:
The faculty member (coach) responsible for students participating in interscholastic athletics such as football, basketball, track and field, baseball and wrestling should evidence knowledge about the medical aspects of sports activities, and should continuously be apprised of the latest developments emanating from the medical and training research on sports activities.

and

BE IT FURTHER RESOLVED that the Superintendent of Public Instruction be, and hereby is, directed to distribute this addition to the Guide to all Superintendents and principals in the state, and to encourage and assist local school districts, the OHSAA and other education-related associations or agencies in planning and holding workshops or seminars for the purpose of developing appropriate knowledge and providing information on the latest developments in this field.

CURRENT TRENDS

Sports form one of the bonds which help bring people together. Cozens and Stumpf acknowledge this concept:

> Within a few decades, sports and games have spread over the whole world, leaping barriers of race, religion, and social class. The language of sport is truly universal, and in the sportsman's code there is neither east nor west, neither white nor black, neither exploiter nor exploited.[4]

Although there is not universal agreement with this statement, particularly with the last phrase, there can be no denial of the fact that the growth of interschool athletic programs in the United States has been nothing short of spectacular. And, far from being restricted to the four activities historically associated with this type of program (football, basketball, baseball, and track and field), the list now includes such diverse sports as field hockey, water polo, gymnastics, bowling, curling, softball, volleyball, lacrosse, and synchronized swimming.

The inclusion of such activities as field hockey and softball is reflective of the phenomenal growth of interschool athletic programs for girls and women. As sociocultural concepts regarding female athletic prowess and femininity change and as research repudiates what were once considered undesirable physiological and psychological effects of competition on females, opportunities for girls to compete have increased even more dramatically than for boys. No doubt, however, the most significant factor in such growth is Title IX of the Education Amendments of 1972 whose final regulation went into effect in July 1975. Insofar as sports programs are concerned, two major substantive provisions of the implementing regulations define the basic responsibility of all schools to provide equal opportunities for athletic participation to both sexes. One of these (Section 86.41) prohibits discrimination on the basis of sex in the conduct of any varsity, club, or intramural program in an educational institution; the other (Section 86.37c) mandates equal opportunity for both sexes in the provision of athletic scholarships. It is necessary to recognize that the regulations for the implementation of Title IX do not indicate

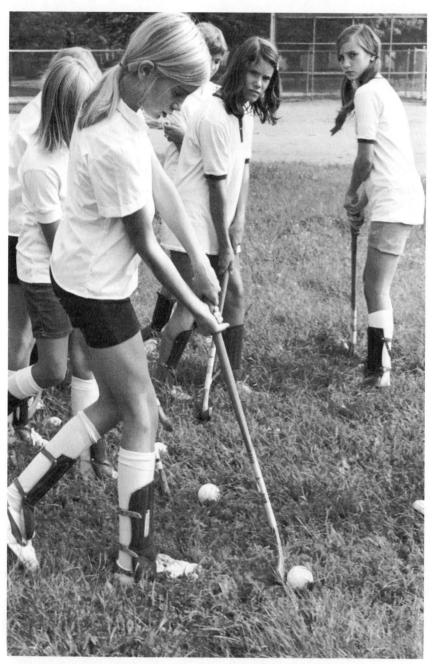

Field hockey, a popular interscholastic sport for girls. Photo courtesy of the Ohio Association for Health, Physical Education and Recreation.

that *equal* treatment means *identical* treatment. Instead schools must offer activities and levels of competition which accommodate the sports interests and abilities of both males and females and there must be equity in providing equipment and supplies, opportunities for coaching, and scheduled practice sessions and games. Separate teams are allowed in those sports involving sufficient body contact to be possibly injurious to the female. The fact that a school sponsors a varsity program for boys in a sport such as football does not necessitate that the same activity be offered for girls so long as the girls are provided the opportunity to compete in a comparable sport such as field hockey or soccer. If, however, a school sponsors a team in those activities which do not involve body contact, such as golf, tennis, swimming, or track and field, it must either provide a team for each sex or allow either sex to try out for the single team. Insofar as athletic scholarships are concerned, the regulations do not require identical sums to be allocated to both sexes nor do they mandate any sort of ratio or fixed percentages in such allocation. "Reasonableness," the thrust of that section of Title IX which deals with athletic scholarships, rests on a concept that the critical factor in determining the allocation of scholarship monies is the *degree* of interest and participation of male and female students. Although the final chapter on the effects of Title IX remains to be written, it seems safe to predict that history will record that this piece of legislation had a far-reaching impact on the development of competitive athletic programs for girls and women.[5]

The fact that agencies sponsoring competitive athletic programs are not limited to educational institutions presents some distinctive problems, not the least of which are questions of standards and leadership. However, there seems to be genuine concern among the various sponsoring agencies about improving programs for the welfare of all participants, so one can be optimistic about the effects of competition.

Problems germane to Olympic competition must be solved and the age-old question of amateurism answered. Reasonable people, truly interested in sport and its congruent values and diligent in their attack on such problems, should be able to provide workable, equitable solutions.

The problems connected with interschool athletic competition, especially at the high school level, are quite varied, and efforts to solve them must consist of more than mere discussion. A solution that seems to promise the greatest likelihood of success in overcoming questionable athletic practices is the trend toward required certification of all coaches. To be certified, a coach must have more than a teaching degree. He or she must have taken courses covering the medical aspects of sports and the psychological and sociological foundations of coaching, and must have become thoroughly grounded in specific game skills.

Curricula which prepare trainers and athletic administrators are also being introduced into American colleges. Since many sports are inherently dangerous, it would be well to have qualified medical personnel at all games and practice sessions, but this is obviously impossible. Greater attention is therefore being paid to the qualifications of trainers, and courses are being prescribed which should enable them to handle most injuries competently.

The area of administration in athletics is no longer just a haphazard arrangement of "promoting" a faithful coach or "kicking upstairs" an unsuccessful one. A recent study in this area points out that most athletic administrators consider a master's degree essential and that courses included in such a degree should cover, in addition to physical education, such things as the science and philosophy of administration, accounting, public relations, management, psychology, and public speaking.[6] Since it is universally accepted that the quality of leadership determines the quality of the program, specific preparation for athletic administrators cannot help being efficacious.

Problems at the intercollegiate level are even more complex and more numerous. Basically, however, they are merely magnifications of problems at the high school level, and since most prospective physical educator-coaches will not commence their careers at the college level, we will give no special attention to these problems here. Those interested will find a cogent treatment of the entire spectrum of intercollegiate athletics in the recently published *Administration of Athletics in Colleges and Universities.*[7]

Like all other educational endeavors, the interschool athletic program is experiencing a new kind of problem as a new generation of student athletes enters the picture. Most boys and girls still have an interest in sports as well as a desire to participate in them; however, many will no longer accept what they consider infringements on their freedom in order to be members of varsity squads. Such things as length of hair, extremely restrictive training rules and regulations, and unquestioning attitude seem immaterial to many present-day athletes in their pursuit of athletic excellence. Consequently, if faced by the achetypal coach who refuses to change procedures, many potentially good athletes simply drop out of the program, preferring instead to be true to their own convictions. It seems that a required background for all coaches in the behavioral sciences would help to alleviate this situation.

There are many other problem areas in athletics, and there are just as many proposed solutions to them. Not the least of the problems is, of course, financing. Theoretically, if a program of athletics is educational, it ought to be financed as are other educational endeavors; that is, it should be completely subsidized by boards of education. Although this goal seems unattainable under the present tax structure for supporting public schools, it is worth fighting for, and we can hope that all educators will join in the struggle to guarantee such subsidy for all cocurricular programs.

CLUB SPORTS

Modern athletics had their beginnings, at least partially, in club sports. In the late 1800s and early 1900s sports clubs in this country experienced rapid and uncontrolled growth, marked by a lack of proper equipment, adequate financing, and proper standards. As a result, faculty and administrative controls were mandated, controls which seem to have fostered a subsequent turning away from clubs toward an emphasis on a varsity program.

In the intervening years student groups interested in a particular sport have on occasion applied for varsity status. Often, in order to be assured of sustained interest and proper financing, administrators demand that such groups function first on a club sport basis.

This decade has experienced a rebirth of the club sports movement due in large part to the unfortunate fact that lack of sufficient funding has caused curtailment of varsity programs and thus many students are deprived of opportunities to participate in sports of their choosing. Students now have a greater voice in the determination of how monies which are earmarked for extracurricular activities are spent, and those student interested in nonvarsity or club sports are demanding a fair share of financing.

Club sports fulfill the need for those who are not interested in a highly organized activity with stringent training rules and time restrictions. They also fulfill the needs of those who cannot qualify on varsity eligibility standards because they carry too few course credits, take quarters or semesters away from campus, or are graduate students.

Although sports clubs offer many excellent opportunities for participation in a great variety of activities which need not be scheduled years in advance, they also present the same problems as did the original clubs. Among these are the problems of student behavior, financing which ensures the availability of proper equipment, and possible health and safety problems. The last requires that attention be given to the physical condition of those seeking to participate as well as to the health care of those who are injured in the process. Labeling an activity "club" rather than "varsity" does not reduce the possibility of injuries in such sports as rugby, soccer, or karate.

Sports clubs demand the administration and supervision of a professional—a trained individual, whether a physical educator, recreator, or an athletic administrator—although the sponsors of clubs may be interested and responsible individuals from other fields. The club movement has much to offer. In order to ensure maximum effectiveness, it should be properly cultivated.

SUMMARY

Play is our heritage and as such is universally accepted; yet a long established resistance to organized programs of competitive athletics is also a heritage.[8] Adjustment of diverse viewpoints depends on the efforts of reasonable, principled men and women to define acceptable and justifiable goals for interschool athletic programs, work untiringly to achieve them, and refuse to yield to pressures which would destroy them. Oberteuffer cites reasons for alarm about the future of athletic programs, and he states that it will take an organized effort to "stem the tide of anti-morality and anti-intellectualism" presently engulfing school athletics.[9] It is hoped that some of the points brought out in this chapter will motivate all those interested in physical education and athletics to explore intelligently and scientifically the contributions which sports can make to the education of all boys and girls and then to develop programs that will ensure such contributions.

STUDENT PROJECTS

1. Survey the schools in the immediate area to determine the following:
   a) How many elementary schools sponsor interschool competition? In what sports? How many junior high schools?
   b) Are such programs conducted for both boys and girls?
   c) At the senior high school level: (1) How many sports are there in the interschool program? (2) How are they financed? How many activities are self-supporting? Which ones? (3) Compare the program for girls to the program for boys.
2. Interview coaches to determine what they consider the greatest problems in interscholastic athletics.
3. How is the girls' intercollegiate athletic program at your university financed? If financed differently than the boys' program, why?
4. Interview principals, coaches, and athletes to get an evaluation of the effects of Title IX on the interscholastic athletic program.
5. Interview professors representative of a cross section of disciplines to get their reactions to the value of intercollegiate athletic programs.
6. How does the conduct of interschool athletic programs in the United States differ from that of the same type of program in selected foreign countries?

GLOSSARY OF TERMS

Athletics   That part of the total physical education program which centers around interschool or intercollegiate sports participation.

Varsity   A highly select group of players who receive extra coaching and who participate in prescheduled athletic contests.

State High School Athletic Association   That body in a particular state to whom the State Board of Education delegates the responsibility for the conduct of interscholastic athletic programs.

Intramurals   A program of recreational activities carried on within the school. These activities may or may not be competitive and may or may not be athletic.

Extramurals The extension of the intramural program to include more than one school. For example, all intramural winners from one school may compete against the winners from another school.

Sports days A program of competition in one or more activities in which two or more schools are involved and school identity is maintained.

Play day A program similar to a sports day, except that school identity is *not* maintained. Competing teams are selected from representatives of all participating schools.

REFERENCES

1. Howard J. Savage, *American College Athletics*, Bulletin 23 (New York: Carnegie Foundation for the Advancement of Teaching, 1929).
2. Clifford Fagan, "Values in Interscholastic Sports," in *Values in Sports, Report of a National Conference* (Washington: American Association for Health, Physical Education and Recreation, 1963), pp. 11–12.
3. "State Board of Education Resolution," *The Ohio High School Athlete* **30** (February 1971), p. 123. Reprinted with permission.
4. Frederick W. Cozens and Florence Stumpf, *Sports in American Life* (Chicago: University of Chicago Press, 1953), p. 3.
5. U.S. Department of Health, Education and Welfare. *Final Title IX Regulation Implementing Education Amendments of 1972*. Washington, D.C.: United States Government Printing Office, June 1975.
6. Fredric W. Schuett, "A Comparison of Recommended Duties and Preparations of College Athletic Directors with Present Practices," Master's thesis, Kent State University, 1968.
7. National Association of College Directors of Athletics and Division of Men's Athletics, American Association for Health, Physical Education and Recreation, ed. Edward S. Stietz, *Administration of Athletics in Colleges and Universities* (Washington: National Educational Association, 1971).
8. Edward J. Shea and Elton E. Wieman, *Administrative Policies for Intercollegiate Athletics* (Springfield, Ill.: Charles C Thomas, 1967), p. 3.
9. Delbert Oberteuffer, "On Learning Values Through Sport," *Quest* **1** (December 1963), pp. 23–29.

SELECTED READINGS

AAHPER. *Complying with Title IX*. Washington, D.C.: The Alliance, 1976.

Boyle, Robert H. *Sport—Mirror of American Life*. Boston: Little, Brown, 1963.

Coutts, Curtis A. "Freedom in Sport." *Quest* **10** (May 1968), pp. 68–71.

Division for Girls' and Women's Sports and Division of Men's Athletics. *Values in Sports*. Washington: American Association for Health, Physical Education and Recreation, National Education Association, 1963.

Educational Policies Commission, National Education Association. *School Athletics*. Washington: National Education Association, 1954.

Frost, Reuben, and Sims, E. J., eds. *Development of Human Values Through Sports.* Washington, D.C.: AAHPER, 1974.

Gerber, Ellen et al. *The American Woman in Sport.* Reading, Mass.: Addison-Wesley, 1974.

Hein, Fred V. "Why Some Boys Should Stay Off the Team." *Today's Health* (August 1967), pp. 71–72.

Kroll, Walter. "Psychological Scaling of Proposed Title IX Guidelines." *Research Quarterly* **47**:3 (October 1976), pp. 548–553.

Loy, John W. "The Nature of Sport: A Definitional Effort." *Quest* **10** (May 1968), pp. 1–15.

McIntosh, Peter C. *Sport in Society.* London: C. A. Watts, 1963.

National Association of College Directors of Athletics and Division of Men's Athletics, American Association for Health, Physical Education and Recreation. Edited by Edward S. Stietz. *Administration of Athletics in Colleges and Universities.* Washington: National Educational Association, 1971.

Resick, Matthew C., and Erickson, C. E. *Intercollegiate and Interscholastic Athletics for Men and Women.* Reading, Mass.: Addison-Wesley, 1975.

Resick, Matthew C.; Seidel, Beverly L.; and Mason, James. *Modern Administrative Practices in Physical Education and Athletics.* Reading, Mass.: Addison-Wesley, 1970.

Sanborn, Marion, and Hartman, Betty. *Issues in Physical Education.* Philadelphia: Lea & Febiger, 1970.

Savage, Howard J. *American College Athletics,* Bulletin 23. New York: Carnegie Foundation for the Advancement of Teaching, 1929.

Scott, Harry A. *Competitive Sports in Schools and Colleges.* New York: Harper, 1951.

Scott, Jack. *Athletics of Athletes.* Hayward, Calif.: Quality Printing Service, 1969.

Shea, Edward J., and Wieman, Elton E. *Administrative Policies for Intercollegiate Athletics.* Springfield, Ill.: Charles C Thomas, 1967.

Shecter, Leonard. *The Jocks.* Indianapolis: Bobbs-Merrill, 1969.

Sheehan, Thomas J. "Sport: The Focal Point of Physical Education." *Quest* **10** (May 1968), pp. 59–67.

Stoke, Harold W. "College Athletics, Education or Show Business?" *Atlantic Monthly* (March 1954), pp. 46–50.

Stone, Gregory P. "American Sports: Play and Displays." *Chicago Review* **9** (Fall 1955), pp. 83–100.

Part III
Physical Education
and
Allied Fields
of Study

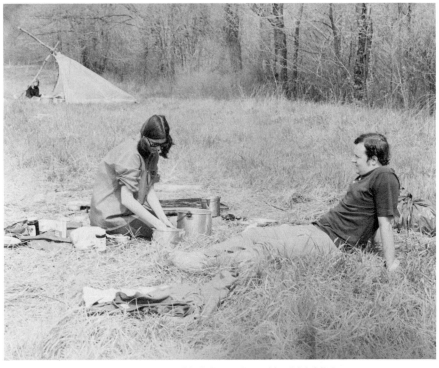

Recreational activity, an added dimension of healthful living.
Photo courtesy of Department of Recreation, Kent State University.

Part III
Physical Education
and
Allied Fields
of Study

Chapter 11
Relationship of Physical Education to Recreation

To be able to fill leisure intelligently is the last product of civilization.

BERTRAND RUSSELL

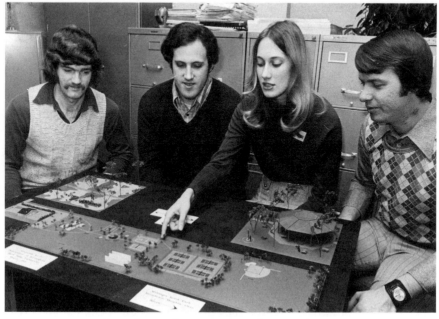

A good recreation program requires attention to
facilities planning. Photo courtesy of Department of Recreation,
Kent State University.

R ECREATION has only recently taken its place among the professions. It has become a profession in part because of the needs of an increasing world population: a decrease in free recreative space, an increase in nonworking hours, and an increase in life expectancy for the general population.

Formerly the various branches of recreation were taught and administered within other areas of specialization. Physical and sports activities were taught by physical educators, nature study by conservationists, and painting by artists. Little or no coordination existed between the different groups which were serving the recreational needs of people. Municipal recreation seemed to have very little in common with park management. Fortunately, that lack of coordination has largely disappeared. Rapid means of transportation now bring the city recreation program to the parks. The city, which controls the water systems for use as designated by the water department, is at times forced to open lakes and reservoirs for recreational uses. The administration of these water activities may be entrusted to the city's recreation department.

As needs for recreation specialists increased, colleges and universities began to offer preparatory courses in recreation leadership. Because the personnel involved were lacking in expertise, such programs were often multidisciplinary. The multidisciplinary pattern was thus a product of necessity, but it proved to be a strong advantage because it drew on the talents found in the related fields of biology, geology, physical education, and astronomy—to name just a few.

Later, divergent groups such as park managers, city recreation directors, industrial recreation directors, and others began to hold joint meetings to form professional associations. Strength of purpose, program, and personnel followed. Recreation no longer needs to depend on other fields to train its personnel although it will always continue to call on the expertise available in selected areas of preparation.

The fact that even professional educators tend to think of the fields of physical education and recreation as synonymous contributes to the confusion of terminology discussed in Chapter 1. A similar problem is that recreation is at times interpreted to mean solely "play," leisure time, or physical activity. Although each one of these interpretations is correct in some degree, none suffices as a definition of recreation as a field of study or discipline.

There are a number of definitions of play and various theories on why animals, including humans, play. Some of the theories propose, for example, that children play because they have surplus energy, that they are reliving in play the history of the human race, that they instinctively know what they will do in later life, that the basic drive to play is similar to the drive to seek food, that children play because of their social contacts with others. There seems to be some foundation to each theory, and yet no one is adequate by itself, and most of them are unable to explain the play patterns of large segments of the human race.

Since play may be considered part of recreation, it may have some of the characteristics of recreation, but no definition of play is completely satisfying as a definition of recreation. The same limitation applies to leisure, which can be defined as "the unobligated hours available after caring for employment or the activities mandatory for self-maintenance."[1] Again, leisure time is part of the recreation whole, not synonymous with it. Carlson, Deppe, and McClean defined recreation as "any enjoyable leisure experience in which the participant voluntarily engages and from which he receives immediate satisfaction."[2] Most writers on recreation prefer to define it in terms of the characteristics which mark recreative activities.

THE CHARACTERISTICS OF RECREATION

Recreation encompasses many activities, from those of a quiet, sedentary type to vigorous contact sports. This fact influences the philosophers among the recreation specialists to shy away from a short and concise definition of the discipline and to favor one that combines a number of descriptive characteristics.

> Recognizing that the task of the recreation professional is a varied and complex one, and that he may appear in many different lights to different observers, it is appropriate at this point to examine the meaning of the term "recreation" itself. Most people—including many professionals in this field—feel they have a fairly good idea of what this is. But, when they are pinned down and asked to define the word, the results are likely to be contradictory and confused.[3]

When one peruses the literature in the recreation field, the similarities in the descriptions of the *characteristics* of recreation become very pronounced. Among those most often listed are the following characteristics.

1. *A recreational activity must be voluntary.* As soon as a person is forced into an activity by pressure of individuals or peer groups, it is no longer considered recreational in nature.

2. *To be recreational, an activity must take place during leisure time.* The fact that one enjoys his or her occupation does not make it recreational. Occasionally, however, skill in a creational activity may lead to an occupation, such as art or professional sport.

3. *There must in fact be activity, not mere passive diversion.* Daydreaming, taking a nap, and sitting on a park bench may be restful, but they are not recreative in nature, as are such quiet activities as bridge and painting.

4. *To be recreational, an activity must be intrinsically enjoyable.* Since it is voluntary and takes place during free time, no one should participate in an activity he or she doesn't enjoy. Recreational activities are not performed for social acceptance or reward.

5. *To be recreational, an activity must have social acceptance.* Stealing hub caps might well fulfill some of the criteria, but the practice is not accepted by society in general.

6. *To be recreational, an activity must provide a change from one's usual activity.* Professional painters cannot paint "for recreation" within the definition of that term, although they may indeed enjoy painting (see 2 above). Neither would a professional golfer playing nontournament golf be considered to be participating in recreational activity.

7. *To be recreational, an activity must not be related to personal or family maintenance.* Eating, grooming, and housekeeping are thus excluded as recreational activities except under circumstances limited enough to be insignificant.

8. *To be recreational, an activity must permit creative responses.* Although regimentation may be necessary in some recreational activities, it must not be of a degree to stifle creative individual responses to the problems presented in the activities.

THE NEED FOR RECREATION

From the earliest of primitive times, people hunted and fished for food to survive, and in such pursuits they protected themselves from attack. Yet even in those times, they amused themselves with objects of play. Furthermore, when it was no longer necessary to hunt and fish for survival, it was still done for the pleasure found in the activity, and hence recreation was born. The history of recreational activities parallels that of physical education, as described in Chapter 2, and it is sometimes impossible to separate the two. Recreation has always been needed, but the reasons for the needs have varied throughout history. A review of the needs, especially those of the present day, seems to be in order.

1. *The expansion of leisure.* Except among members of the ruling classes in Western Europe, the expansion of leisure occurred only after the invention of industrial machines. In the early days of the Industrial Revolution, some machines produced more goods but actually increased the length of the working day.

The Greeks, on the other hand, had taken time for their recreative pursuits, and so had the Romans. During the time of Nero, the Romans were reported to have had 159 holidays that were devoted to spectacles. Unfortunately, most of the Romans were merely spectators, and the slaves in combat could hardly be considered as engaging in recreation! The period after World War I marked the beginning of the reduction of the workweek. After the Great Depression the workweek was further reduced, either because of the economics of supply and demand or because of legislation enacted to bring the crisis to a solution. During that period the rise of a united labor force was the greatest single factor in effecting the reduction of the workweek—a process that continues even today. A workweek shorter than 40 hours is no longer a dream. The two-day weekend has long been a reality. In many occupations the midweek half-day break is common practice. This additional released time will make demands on recreation facilities. A recent suggestion that reservations be required before admission to our national parks is one way in which to cope with the hordes that descend on them at critical periods of the year.

Recreation programs must be planned to meet the increase in leisure in ways other than the sedentary pursuits of radio and television.

2. *The rise of urban centers.* When America was predominantly rural, the process of earning a living demanded long hours, but opportunities for recreation abounded. There were fish to catch, game to hunt, mountains to climb, and fresh streams to swim. Groups gathered together for such social occasions as plowing and husking bees, log tossing and rolling, and the combative sports of men. As time passed, however, buildings rose, the streets became hard, and people moved inward and upward. Land has become increasingly expensive and decreasingly available for leisure time play or recreation. In this setting, people run machines, mostly in a sedentary position. There is certainly a paradox in the fact that people work with machines for the better life, and yet keep decreasing the space in which we can enjoy the fruits of our labors. We need now to replace the opportunities for recreation in the setting we have created for ourselves or to be transported away from it for our leisure.

3. *The changing social structure.* In the past the family unit was the center of most recreation activities. Changes that have been evolving for many years are due to changes in life patterns, including the change from home-centered to business-centered employment. The commuting father placed the burden for family recreation on the mother. Because of the shortage of labor during World War II, the working mother also abrogated much of the responsibility. The trend still continues in this direction, and only time will tell what the present Women's Liberation movement will bring. Some agency must then fill the void and provide leadership to the children in this setting.

Another social factor deserving consideration is the need of the aged for recreation. The time gap between either forced or voluntary retirement and death is increasing steadily. Retired persons who have worked hard all their lives to support themselves and rear their families seek pleasurable ways in which to spend their golden years. They are in need of adequate recreation. Meyer, Brightbill, and Sessoms have listed the needs of the aging in the following manner.

1. The need to be considered as a real part of the community.
2. The need to occupy much expanded free time in more satisfactory ways.

3. The need to render some socially useful service.

4. The need to enjoy normal companionships.

5. The need for recognition as an individual.

6. The need to have opportunity for self-expression.

7. The need for a sense of achievement (tied up with number 5).

8. The need to feel free to slow down on work or activities.

9. The need to have health protection and care.

10. The need for suitable mental stimulation.

11. The need for suitable living arrangements.

12. The need for wholesome family relationships.

13. The need for spiritual satisfaction.[4]

THE VALUES OF RECREATION

When one discusses the values that accrue from participation in most disciplines or professions, the possibility of making unsubstantiated claims becomes real. Recreation does not profess to be a cure for juvenile delinquency or the salvation of the aged. It may contribute to both, however. Among the values associated with recreation in its many aspects are the following.

1. There are opportunities to develop physically through muscular activity. Some activities, such as handball and swimming, develop the

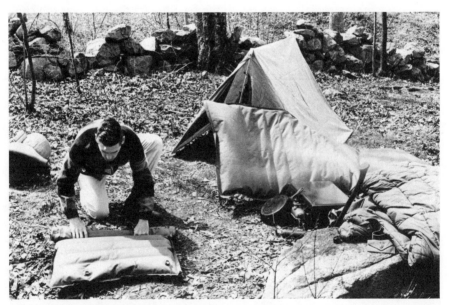

Backpacking and orienteering are popular recreational activities. Photo courtesy of Department of Recreation, Kent State University.

cardiovascular system, some develop strength, and others help develop coordination. The degree of contribution usually depends on the intensity of the activity and the time devoted to it.

2. There are opportunities to enhance the educative process through recreational activities. Play permits children to investigate the immediate surroundings, and solutions are often determined by trial and error. Activities such as photography permit the participant to learn about the processes necessary for the development of pictures.

3. There are opportunities to discover innate creativity through exposure to the fine arts. Activities such as painting, music, dramatics, and gymnastics permit the participants to express themselves in their relationships with their world.

4. There are opportunities to engage in and improve social interaction in acceptable situations. Camping presents many opportunities for people of different states and different countries to get to know one another in an informal and friendly atmosphere. Bowling and golf leagues permit people of all ages to unite for a common goal. For young children, the opportunity of learning to compete under socially acceptable conditions is essential. The sacrifices one must make for the common good and the cooperation necessary for success can be imparted through these activities.

5. There are opportunities for a change in pace from one's everyday life. No matter how enjoyable one's work is, there is a need to get away from it occasionally. Even people who make a living doing what they enjoy most, derive benefits from detaching themselves from it. Painters who love to paint and professional golfers or baseball players certainly do have enjoyable vocations, and yet in the late stages of a long season, they need a change. There are enough forms of recreation to satisfy the needs of most people for change.

6. There are opportunities for individuals to obtain the satisfaction and pleasure of a personal achievement. The unbounded enjoyment of leisure time might be the greatest value of them all. People can set their own goals. A mountain climbed, a trout caught, a tent pitched, or a ball struck can be sheer joy to one who has never had such an experience. To another such joy may come from a first sketch in a drawing class or a simple finesse in bridge. That is what recreation is all about.

HOW RECREATION IS ORGANIZED AND ADMINISTERED TO MEET NEEDS AND VALUES

Since recreation activities range widely—for example, from mountain climbing to collecting sea shells—there is no one organizational pattern which can suffice for all types of recreation available in the United States today. The following paragraphs explain briefly the administrative responsibilities of the principal areas of recreation.

Community recreation department. A recreation department that is an arm of the formal community government gets its financial support from tax sources, general funds, or funds raised by special levies. It may or may not be connected with the school system. Since it gets its money directly from the people, the department does not ordinarily compete for the dollar with other units. It provides low-cost recreation for all of the citizens of the community by utilizing existing buildings and outdoor areas. The necessity of maintaining separate staffs and facilities may be considered a disadvantage.

School-centered recreation. When community recreation is centered in the local school system, the existing facilities are more readily available. Utilization time of school buildings is increased. There is also a ready staff available to run the facilities. In this situation, however, recreation is competing with the school for money. Whenever a conflict of schedules develops, it is usually the recreation program that is altered. Furthermore, participants may feel that recreation in a sense becomes an extension of the school day—to the detriment of a real feeling of recreation.

School and community recreation. A combined organization offers the advantages of both of the separated systems, especially in the small to medium-sized communities that cannot afford separate sets of facilities. In some larger cities (for example, Cleveland, Ohio) it also works very well.

State and federal governments. Through their systems of forests and parks, both the state and federal governments provide a wide range of recreation activities as part of their services. Camping, hunting, fishing, hiking, horseback riding, swimming, and golf, which are included in such programs, are usually low-cost activities. Some the available park lands and forests remain fixed in extent, the existing facilities are now becoming overcrowded. Areas once considered remote are now readily accessible by modern means of transportation.

City government. In addition to specifically including recreation departments with their structures, many cities provide related facilities for recreation purposes. Libraries, zoos, concert halls, and theaters expand a city's recreation possibilities. Some subdivisions within the city are planning recreation services during the development of the area along with such standard items as sewers, sidewalks, and roads.

Industrial recreation. Most large, modern business organizations now provide recreation programs for their staffs and employees. World War II programs proved so successful in both improving employee morale and increasing production that recreation leaders are now considered indispensable members of business firms. Programs are limited only by the imagination of those in charge. Music groups, theater, athletic teams, and craft classes are found in many such programs.

Geriatric centers. Among the more interesting recent developments in the recreation field is the provision of recreation for senior citizens. Most of these people are retired, and they are seeking worthwhile recreation activities. States such as Florida, California, and Arizona have been particularly concerned with this area of recreation because large numbers of older citizens have moved to those states. Retirement villages have sprung up where retired persons enjoy common interests.

Commercial recreation. During periods of affluence, commercial recreation facilities are constructed at a very rapid rate. Golf courses, bowling alleys, tennis clubs, ski resorts, archery ranges, and trampoline areas are examples. Adding these new facilities to the older fishing and hunting camps and seaside resorts, one can see the impact of recreation activities. Though often criticized by the recreation professional, these resorts must be good to survive. Programs must be well conducted and interesting.

Fraternal organizations and service clubs. The American Legion has sponsored a youth baseball program for many years. The Fraternal Order of Police sponsors the PAL program, which provides organized activities for needy youngsters. Little need be said for the long-standing programs of both the YMCA and the YWCA; indeed, in historical terms, it is difficult to separate physical education in the United States and the development of the YMCA movement.

THE PHYSICAL EDUCATOR AND RECREATION

Although presently the disciplines of physical education and recreation have a great deal of autonomy, at one time the source of personnel for recreation was primarily the physical education schools. Recreation became an avocation or even the second occupation of the physical educator. During this period, most recreational activities were mainly physical in nature. With the extension of recreation to include a wide variety of activities and the development of a separate philosophy, the profession of recreation began to develop its own personnel with specialties in community recreation, industrial recreation, recreational therapy, and park management. The curricula at a number of institutions reflected this change at both the undergraduate and graduate levels. Recreation has come into its own as a profession. The physical educator still has a place in recreation, but he or she is usually a specialist in playground direction, much as the art instructor is a specialist in, say, painting.

Since many high school students do not go on to higher education, the physical education program should include some of the activities which the students can use throughout adult life. The Lifetime Sports Education Project has been instrumental in having such sports as tennis, golf, bowling, trap-shooting, archery, and bait and fly casting added to the curriculum in many schools throughout the country. This goal has been achieved mainly by offering a series of workshops and clinics to teachers in various parts of the country. Most have been conducted by well-known experts in the particular sports and sponsored jointly by the Lifetime Sports Education Project and the state or national professional organizations.

The job opportunities in recreation are excellent. There will be a shortage of personnel in the foreseeable future. Most of the areas mentioned in the preceding section on administration are shorthanded. In addition, the colleges and universities that offer courses in recreation are in need of key personnel. As the general population increases, continued periods of prosperity and a general increase in leisure will continue to compound the situation.

STUDENT PROJECTS

1. Visit in a group and/or research the different types of recreation programs (municipal, industrial, private, etc.) and report your findings to the class.
2. Investigate the occupational opportunities in the recreation field.

GLOSSARY OF TERMS

Leisure   "The unobligated hours available after caring for employment or the activities mandatory for self-maintenance." (Carlson, Deppe, and McClean)

Recreation   "Any enjoyable leisure experience in which the participant voluntarily engages and from which he receives immediate satisfactions." (Carlson, Deppe, and McClean)

Play   Voluntary participation in a game activity, either educational or recreational in nature.

REFERENCES

1. Reynold E. Carlson, Theodore R. Deppe, and Janet R. McClean, *Recreation in American Life,* (Belmont, Calif.: Wadsworth, 1936), p. 6.
2. Ibid., p. 7.
3. From *Recreation Today: Program Planning and Leadership,* by Richard Kraus. Copyright © 1966 by Meredith Publishing Company, p. 5. Reprinted by permission of Appleton-Century-Crofts, Educational Division, Meredith Corporation.

4. Harold D. Meyer, Charles K. Brightbill, and H. Douglas Sessoms, *Community Recreation,* 4th ed. (Englewood Cliffs, N.J.: Prentice-Hall, 1969), pp. 337–338.

SELECTED READINGS

Brantley, Herbert, and Sessoms, H. Douglas, eds. *Recreation Issues and Perspectives.* Columbia, S.C.: Wing, 1969, pp. 111–167.

Carlson, Reynold E.; Deppe, Theodore R.; and McClean, Janet R. *Recreation in American Life.* Belmont, Calif.: Wadsworth, 1963.

Danford, Howard G. *Creative Leadership in Recreation.* Boston: Allyn and Bacon, 1964.

Kleindienst, Viola, and Weston, Arthur. *Intramural and Recreation Programs for Schools and Colleges.* New York: Appleton-Century-Crofts, 1964.

Kraus, Richard. *Recreation and Leisure in Modern Society.* New York: Appleton-Century-Crofts, 1971.

Meyer, Harold D.; Brightbill, Charles K.; and Sessoms, H. Douglas. *Community Recreation,* 4th ed. Englewood Cliffs, N.J.: Prentice-Hall, 1969.

Nash, Jay B. *Philosophy of Recreation and Leisure.* Dubuque, Iowa: Wm. C. Brown, 1960.

———. *Recreation: Pertinent Readings.* Dubuque, Iowa: Wm. C. Brown, 1965.

———. *The Organization and Administration of Playgrounds and Recreation.* New York: A. S. Barnes, 1936.

Neumeyer, Martin H., and Neumeyer, Esther S. *Leisure and Recreation.* New York: A. S. Barnes, 1936.

Sessoms, Douglas H.; Meyer, Harold S.; and Brightbill, Charles K. *Leisure Services, the Organized Recreation and Park System.* Englewood Cliffs, N.J.: Prentice-Hall, 1971.

Chapter 12
Relationships of Physical Education with Health Education as a Profession

It is better to lose health like a spendthrift than to waste it like a miser.

BALZAC

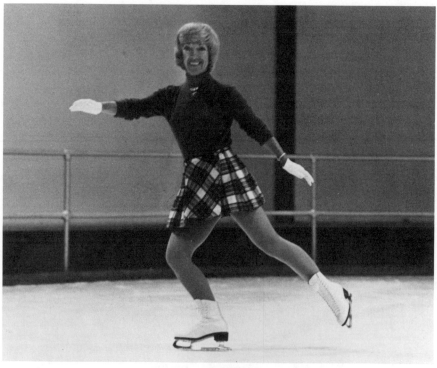

Good health enables an individual to participate in vigorous activities.

"HEALTH and physical education"

"HEALTH and physical education" have been used as one term so long in different settings of education that it is difficult to identify them as separate and distinct disciplines. Many states still certify teachers of "health and physical education," and departments within the school structure are frequently so titled. It seems appropriate to examine the reasons for both the earlier pattern of combination and the growing tendency to separate the two into distinct disciplines.

A SHORT HISTORY OF HEALTH EDUCATION

Although health and the effects on it of the environment figured in writings in Colonial America, the subject was not treated as a separate entity in the schools of that period. William A. Alcott (1798–1859) is considered the father of school health education because he wrote on the school environment and necessary health services. Even in his day, however, health was linked to physical education, as the writings of Horace Mann indicate. As a result of Alcott's efforts, Massachusetts became the first state to require by law the teaching of health (1850). Harvard College had initiated a course in hygiene by 1818.

During the latter stages of the nineteenth century, the "marriage" of health and physical education became almost complete, probably because: (1) heads of departments of physical education were mostly medical doctors, (2) the objectives had much in common, and (3) the curricular needs of both were met, to a great extent, in common courses.

This union continued well into the twentieth century, although Thomas Wood and others were disturbed by the lack of attention devoted to health education. There were organizations promoting health education, including some within the federal government, but health continued to play a secondary role in departments of health and physical education and in professional associations. Meanwhile, health *services* were fully accepted and played a major role in the school.

Until after World War I, no teacher training institution offered a major in health education. The first major program was established in Teachers College, Columbia University, in the year 1920–1921. World War II became the real turning point, however. Because of the exploding knowledge in health education and the pressures from health-allied organizations, a number of institutions began offering separate degrees in health education, including master's and doctor's degrees.

A trend noted in the early 1970s is to distinguish the fields of health education and physical education through separate certification requirements. The day of the joint major at either the undergraduate or the graduate levels has come to an end. Although the two fields still have some common objectives, they will no longer have common facilities or personnel. The discipline of health education has come of age. The effects of the separation on either of the two related fields is a matter of conjecture at this time. In an age of exploding knowledge and specialization, one can hope that both will benefit, but with growing difficulties in the tax support of public schools, both may suffer.

DEFINITIONS AND PURPOSES OF SCHOOL HEALTH EDUCATION

Health is that quality of life which permits us to function at our best within our environment. It has physical, mental, and social implications, which differ in individuals and groups. The necessary level of social and mental health of a student living in a residence hall may have little relevance for a hermit. In a similar sense, the level of physical health and fitness for a bank president is not the same as for a steel worker.

Although health education is ordinarily a joint venture of school and community, this chapter will concern school health education primarily and will refer to community health only when such reference is applicable. In maintaining this approach we recognize nevertheless that the responsibilities for school health education may rest solely with the local health department or jointly with the schools and the local health department. For either organizational pattern, the purposes of the health education program should be the same.

1. To disseminate information to the student concerning health and those factors which have an impact on it. The information may range from the structure of the body to the use of community agencies for the solution of health problems.
2. To initiate a positive health attitude in the student. For example, the student may have adequate knowledge about the problems of smoking or weight control, but a change in attitude may be necessary before he or she will use that knowledge.
3. To influence the student to change his or her behavior now or in the future. In the final analysis, the test of health education is not what people know about the subject, but what they do about it.

It is often assumed that if people acquire knowledge in a certain area, a change in their attitude and behavior in that area will naturally follow. Most of us are examples of the fallacy of this assumption. Indeed, the order may be reversed. A child may respond to a teacher's or mother's "brush your teeth" or "wash your hands" long before understanding dental caries or the germ theory of disease. Then, too, a student with excellent knowledge may be faced with a personal problem that causes an attitudinal change.

In order to achieve the three purposes cited above, health educators organize the health experiences of students into three categories: health instruction, school health services, and the school environment. All three

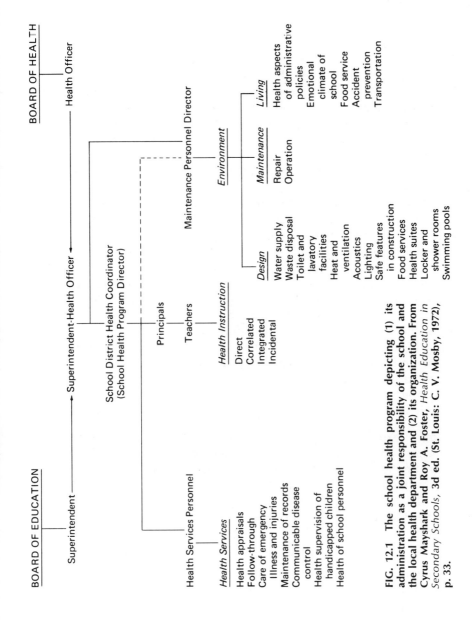

BOARD OF EDUCATION

Superintendent

Superintendent-Health Officer

School District Health Coordinator
(School Health Program Director)

Principals

Teachers

Maintenance Personnel Director

BOARD OF HEALTH

Health Officer

Health Services Personnel

Health Services

Health appraisals
Follow-through
Care of emergency
  Illness and injuries
Maintenance of records
Communicable disease
  control
Health supervision of
  handicapped children
Health of school personnel

Health Instruction

Direct
Correlated
Integrated
Incidental

Environment

Design

Water supply
Waste disposal
Toilet and
  lavatory
  facilities
Heat and
  ventilation
Acoustics
Lighting
Safe features
  in construction
Food services
Health suites
Locker and
  shower rooms
Swimming pools

Maintenance

Repair
Operation

Living

Health aspects
  of administrative
  policies
Emotional
  climate of
  school
Food service
Accident
  prevention
Transportation

FIG. 12.1 The school health program depicting (1) its administration as a joint responsibility of the school and the local health department and (2) its organization. From Cyrus Mayshark and Roy A. Foster, *Health Education in Secondary Schools,* **3d ed. (St. Louis: C. V. Mosby, 1972), p. 33.**

make important contributions to the student's knowledge of health. They will be more fully discussed in the following sections of this chapter. The diagram in Fig. 12.1 shows how the three areas of health education can be arranged for administration in a joint school and community health department.[1]

HEALTH INSTRUCTION

Even though health, historically, was not considered a course in the academic sense of the word, some of what is considered health education was always taught in correlation with other subjects, as part of an integrated unit or project, or incidentally, during the great "teaching moments" which take place as a result of such happenings as tornadoes, hurricanes, earthquakes, or space landings. Under such circumstances, however, the great abundance of exploding health knowledge remained untaught, and serious gaps in health knowledge of students existed. Even with extensive planning, the teaching of health through a series of integrated projects or in correlation with subjects such as biology, physics, and social studies has been found wanting.

Every school needs a concentrated series of courses in health to deal with problems that confront students of different age and grade levels. Although some of these problems (such as acne) are of interest to only one grade or age level, many of the others cross many grade-level lines. The problem of drug abuse, for example, is beginning in the elementary schools and continuing throughout adult life.

The biggest problems confronting the schools are the selection of materials to be taught and the proper introduction and grade placement of such materials. Subjects which formerly were reserved for discussion at the upper secondary grades or college are now topics for study at the junior high schools, and rightly so. Among them are the following.

1. *Human sexuality*. Study begins in the early elementary grades with information about sex-role differences and continues throughout life. Early maturation and dating make the inclusion of proper materials at the junior high school level mandatory. The acceptance of pregnant girls in the total high school program and changes in the obscenity laws create a climate that underscores the need to continue the study of human sexuality.

2. *Drug use and abuse*. Problems relating to drugs are no longer confined to the very few in the lower echelons of society or to the adult age group. Since cases of drug addiction are being discovered in children not yet in their teens, instruction on the dangers involved in drug use must begin at the elementary level before the students are subjected to the pressures of peers to adopt a life-style that includes the use of drugs. Use of and traffic in glue sniffing, marijuana, LSD, and heroin have legal as well as social implications.

The effects of caffeine, alcohol, nicotine, amphetamine, and steroids were discussed in some detail in Chapter 8.

3. *Environmental problems.* The pollution of the air we breathe and the water we drink has become a national emergency because it not only threatens our health but also constitutes aesthetic loss and diminishes recreation opportunities. The pollution of the nation's usable water may result in a severe water shortage in several decades unless the trend is reversed.

Radiation, in addition to polluting the air and water, accumulates in plants and animals, sometimes causing genetic changes in those forms of life. The effects of low-grade radiation are still virtually unknown. The dramatic effects of the "bomb" with its concussions, burns, and cancer-causing qualities are well established.

Pesticides, which were once proclaimed as our saviors, are now suspected of causing a number of illnesses. Governmental agencies are urging caution and restraint in the use of most pesticides, and they have banned some entirely.

The use of food additives and substitutes has created hazards to the health of the user. Such additives and substitutes have been used to make food cheaper, more attractive, less fattening, and more appetizing. Some have been found to contribute to unhealthful conditions, especially as agents that may play a causative part in cancer, and they are now under study.

4. *Mental health.* The promotion of good mental health and the avoidance of mental illness are dealt with at all grade levels in order to emphasize the preventive rather than the curative aspects of this growing problem. Work time lost due to mental illness is among the nation's most critical problems since recovery time is often extensive. For this reason, early detection of minor problems and an emphasis on positive mental health are of crucial importance.

5. *Social and ethical problems.* The legal and ethical problems involved in organ transplants and in the control of the exploding population, for example, pose meaningful questions for both high school and college students. The very definitions of life and death are now being revised.

The topics suggested above, together with more traditional topics, such as rest, exercise, weight control, and consumer education, can make the contents of a relevant curriculum in health education from kindergarten through college vital and exciting. If such a course of study is to have meaning for the student, it must be taught from a psychological or problematical approach rather than from the exclusively physiological, or systems, approach that has been customary in the past. The development of concepts concerning health is more important than the accumulation of knowledge that rapidly becomes outdated.

SCHOOL HEALTH SERVICES

In addition to what the students are taught about health in the formal classroom, many of their experiences in and about the school add to their knowledge and attitudes about health. Since participation in health services is often very personal, a good program may be the principal tool in reaching a student. Although few public schools today can fully qualify, a good health service program should contain the following aspects.

1. *Periodic physical examinations.* Some states require an annual examination of all students attending elementary and secondary schools, but most do not. Where there is no such requirement, a periodic physical should be given four times during a student's schooling: (1) on first entering school, (2) during elementary school, (3) during junior high school, and (4) during senior high school.

At one time physical examinations were conducted on school premises, but at present the usual practice is for the family physician to examine the child and send the results to the school. The change to the physician's examining room should ensure a more thorough examination than could be provided in the school. Equipment is available for any special testing that may be necessary, and complete records are kept on the child's growth and development. Different arrangements, however, must be made for children of needy families.

2. *Special examinations.* There are times other than the periods specified in the preceding paragraph when students will need to be seen by a physician. Athletes in contact sports and other vigorous activities, for example, should have examinations before being allowed to participate in athletics. The heart, lungs, teeth, and tonsils should be examined, and the student should be checked for hernia.

A special examination should also be given to students after a prolonged absence from school because of illness to ensure their readiness to participate in physical education classes or athletics.

3. *Examination follow-up program.* One of the valid criticisms leveled at schools in the past has been the failure to use information gained from physical examinations. In the desire to adhere to the principle of "privileged communication," the results of examinations were "locked away" and seldom referred to. The school should make use of these records in any way that will benefit the student. A physical examination loses part of its value if there is no attempt to correct those deviations from the norm which are correctable. Parents or guardians must be informed about the health status of their children. If the parents cannot afford to have corrections made because of their financial status, referral to an agency that takes care of such matters is in order.

4. *Vaccination and inoculation program.* Although most states have compulsory vaccination and inoculation programs against communicable diseases as a school entrance requirement, schools in the states that do not must formulate their own requirements. The principal communicable diseases are virtually nonexistent in the United States, but they still abound in many parts of the world, and any relaxation of our program could lead to an epidemic. The immunization program in schools is occasionally objected to on the grounds of religious beliefs. Even when exceptions are made in such cases, the communicable diseases can be kept at a nonepidemic level in the student population unless unusual circumstances prevail. Among the diseases for which immunization should be required for school attendance are smallpox, diphtheria, whooping cough, poliomyelitis, tetanus, and measles. Standard immunizations for these diseases, with the possible exception of that for poliomyelitis, do not guarantee lifetime immunity and do require booster shots at specified intervals.

5. *A system of health referrals and health consultations.* Every school system should have a definite policy of dealing with students with health problems, including exclusion from class and exclusion from school. Minor illnesses may be handled by health service personnel, but recurrent or prolonged problems should be referred to the home or a community agency for solution. Exclusion from school sometimes involves legal problems, since the responsibility rests with the school that the student can reach home and that someone will be there when the student arrives. The excluding officer of the school must be sure that these conditions are met before releasing an ill student. All teachers should recognize symptoms in health and behavior that might be significant and refer students exhibiting such symptoms to the health service or counselor. Sight and hearing problems, especially, often develop between the periodic health examinations.

6. *First aid and safety provisions.* Most states have laws requiring each school building to provide a rest and recovery room for students. The room should contain cots, toilets, and lavatories. Since it is not feasible to have a doctor or even a nurse on duty at all times in each building, someone trained and certified in first aid should be readily available. Ideally, all teachers should be certified in first aid procedures.

A plan should be established for handling any type of emergency. The school should require each parent or guardian to complete a form containing pertinent information, including the name of the person to be notified in the event of an emergency. It should list the parent's name and phone number, family physician and phone number, and an alternative person to be notified when a parent cannot be reached, a person who has the legal right to make a decision regarding the child if he or she is sick or injured. A form of this type is shown in Fig. 12.2. Such a form should be readily accessible and near a telephone.

EMERGENCY INFORMATION

Student: Last name	First		Middle initial

1.

Parents or guardians: Last name   Father   Mother

Address   Phone

Parent's emergency number (employer):   Phone

2.   Family physician: Last name   First

Address   Phone

3.   Other physician

4.   In case of emergency, what hospital should be used?

5.   Name of relative or friend who is approved to make   Phone
      decisions in case you cannot be reached.

6.   In case none of the above can be reached, may we have permission to make a decision?

          Yes   No

                                           Signature

FIGURE 12.2

The information it contains must be kept current to be effective. Athletic coaches and intramural directors who stay after school with large numbers of students should have easy access to this information, or they should have their squad members complete similar forms for their own use.

7. *System of screening tests and observations.* Since there may be three or four years between physical examinations, the school system should develop a series of screening procedures. Simple height and weight charts can bring to light deviations from the norm that occur between examinations and that can be investigated before they become serious. When combined with information on body typing, data on height and weight become extremely valuable.

     Vision should be tested each year in the elementary grades. Either the Snellen or the Massachusetts Vision Test can be used. The latter is superior, though a little more costly, since it isolates conditions of farsightedness as well as nearsightedness. The classroom teacher can administer these tests with a minimum of training.

Hearing testing, in which audiometric devices are used, is much more sophisticated than vision testing and requires longer training periods for the tester. Ordinarily, the school speech and hearing therapist does this type of testing.

8. *Health supervision of school personnel.* Where state laws do not require that food handlers have medical examinations, the school board should do so. Since teachers, especially in the elementary schools, have very close contact with students, it should be mandatory that they be free of communicable disease. If nothing else, an annual certification of freedom from tuberculosis should be required. The trend in some states is toward annual examinations of all teachers, paid for by the Board of Education. Some school boards will not release the first salary check until this condition is met. This type of plan is usually a local option of the Board of Education. The state of Maine, for one, requires that all teachers have an annual physical examination.

THE SCHOOL ENVIRONMENT

The location of the physical plant, the relationship of students to teachers, and the nature of the organization for instruction all have an impact on the health of the student. It is essential that the student be provided a most healthful school environment to enhance the learning process. A discussion on the effect of the environment on the student's health and the learning process follows.

1. *The physical environment.* A healthful school environment begins with the location of the school itself. It is difficult to change an established location, and therefore the initial selection of a school site affects students for decades. Is it near railroads, factories, or a main highway? Must most of the students cross the main part of the city to reach it? Is it located in the direction of the future growth of the city?

The disadvantages of old buildings located near noisy factories can be decreased by the use of tree screens between the noise and the school, by careful installation of acoustical tile, and by careful selection of courses to be taught on the noisy and quiet sides of the building.

The school environment also includes the color of the paint on the walls, lighting, humidity and heat, the condition of restrooms, and the adequacy of food services. Laboratories and workshops should be properly vented, and playfields, walks, and building approaches should be properly cared for.

Although most of these problems rest with administration, an alert student body and teaching corps will ensure the maintenance of a healthful school environment. Because of their special expertise, health teachers and administrators have additional responsibility in these areas.

2. *School organization and health.* The manner in which the school day is organized and administered may have at least as much effect on the student as the physical makeup of the school. Among the factors to be considered are the following:

a) *Length of the school day.* It is estimated that the secondary school student now spends more than 1,100 hours a year in school. There are advocates of a longer school day, but with the additional time spent on cocurricular work, most of the student's day is in fact spent in school. The school day is—and should be—gradually lengthened from kindergarten through senior high school, directly in proportion to the decrease in fatigue and the increase in attention span as the student grows older.

b) *Length of class period.* Similar to the problem of school day length is that of class period length. Fatigue and attention span must be considered, and shorter periods in the lower elementary grades permit frequent change in the types of activity. Such change is essential for a proper learning climate at that age level. Periods of 20–30 minutes are common at this level; periods of 40–45 minutes are more usual in the junior and senior high school. At the college level the practice of dog-legging (double period on some days) is necessary to make efficient use of existing space when weekly meetings are variable.

c) *Homework policy.* Some schools have had to initiate a policy of limiting homework assignments to protect the students from demands for unreasonable amounts of work by teachers who seem unaware of the requirements of other disciplines. The school may curtail homework by establishing a time limit per assignment or by restricting homework for each subject to specified days of the week. For instance, English, language, and mathematics teachers may be permitted to give homework on Monday, Wednesday, and Friday, whereas the science, humanities, and social studies teachers are restricted to Tuesday and Thursday.

d) *Curtailment of outside activities.* Often students become involved in too many extra- or cocurricular activities, either by choice or because they are forced by peer or parental pressure to participate. Some schools have restricted students to two or three extracurricular activities. Even though the activities sponsored by the school can be controlled, however, the student may still be subjected to a number of nonschool activities and lessons. The cumulative effect of school work, extracurricular activities, and private lessons may be detrimental to the student. When a student's mental and physical health are endangered by such excesses and pressures, the parents must be notified by the health or counseling services.

e) *Rewards for attendance.* A program of honoring students with perfect attendance records, though understandable in purpose, may actually perform a disservice to the teachers and student body. Some elementary school children come to school with communicable diseases in order to keep their records intact. The attendance certificate becomes of greater significance than their own health or the health of others they come in contact with. The practice of making awards for perfect attendance is fortunately dying out.

f) *Sick-leave program for teachers.* A similar threat to general health may stem from the school's sick-leave policy for teachers. If the teachers must pay for their own substitutes after a maximum number of absences, some will come to school with such communicable diseases as influenza, thus exposing students and other members of the faculty. On the other hand, a program which allows the accumulation of sick days for future use may result in a similar response: the teacher may "save" them for a protracted illness.

g) *Time placement of difficult subjects.* In the self-contained classroom of the elementary school, teachers can arrange the course to meet the needs of the students. They can plan to teach the more difficult subjects during that part of the day when the students are most rested and relaxed, or they can alternate them with recreational types of classes, such as art, music, or physical education. Unfortunately, however, at most large secondary schools, not every student can have a desirable schedule. All subjects are taught during most hours of the school day, and the student must take them when they fit into the schedule and not when they are most fit to take them.

3. *The teacher and student health.* The interpersonal relationships between the teacher and the students within the classroom have an impact on the health of the students. Among the considerations which contribute to student health are the following:

a) *The make-up program following absence.* Frequently the procedures followed in having students make up missed work are in direct contradiction to the practices of good health. Following an illness that necessitated absence from school, students are often inundated with make-up work to complete while they are still recovering. In other words, immediately on their return to school, they are expected to produce more than the healthy students.

b) *Seating arrangements.* Because it is practical (administratively) to follow some ascending or descending alphabetical order in seating students, a teacher may inadvertently place students with sight or hearing problems in positions that may retard their progress in class. Taking attendance, collecting written work, and grading may be facilitated by this arrangement, but students may suffer for it. A proper health service identifies the students with handicaps tactfully and without the knowledge of the other students.

c) *Fear of the teacher or subject matter.* In a class where there is factual fear of physical harm for either poor performance or failure to perform at all, students may suffer impairment of their health. If the teacher uses the technique of ridicule or embarrassment, students may have a similar reaction. When exchanges between teachers and students occur in an atmosphere of mutual respect, stress and tensions are held to a minimum. Leniency in course requirements is not in any sense necessary to achieve this ideal, however. Students may learn to enjoy a difficult subject if they are encouraged whenever they show improvement and progress. Criticism of a student's actions may be offered in the interests of improvement, and creative self-expression is not stifled in a rush to conformity.

d) *Free expression.* Although the demand for student silence in a classroom may impair the learning process, the opposite may also be true. Young children forced to work in the bedlam that surrounds the overpermissive teacher may experience complete mental and physical fatigue at the end of the day. Studies have shown that excessive noise causes physical fatigue among factory workers, and one can reasonably assume the same effect on students.

e) *Overemphasis on one grade or performance.* There are situations in the educational system in which one performance may change the course of a student's educational life. An example is the series of scholarship examinations. Although such practices are common in Europe, no single test or performance should carry sufficient weight to cause extreme tension and frustration among the student body.

OCCUPATIONAL OPPORTUNITIES

The entire field of health sciences is rich in career opportunities which combine the excitement of exploding knowledge and a feeling of service to others. At present and for the foreseeable future, there is a shortage of trained and qualified personnel in most areas of the health sciences, of which health education is a part. Furthermore, with the population increasing and with growing concern for the health needs of everyone, there will certainly be demands for more and more persons to become involved in health education as a career.

One thinks of health educators as being confined to formal educational systems, from the elementary schools to the universities. Far from it! Job opportunities exist in such voluntary health agencies as the American Cancer Society, the National Tuberculosis Association, and others. These organizations, which are supported by voluntary financial contributions and services, employ staff members at the national, state, and local levels. Since each agency is generally concerned with a specific health problem, trained personnel are hired to educate the public concerning that particular problem in an effort to combat or eradicate it.

There are also many opportunities in "official health agencies," the tax-supported arms of local, state, and federal government. Examples are city and county health departments, state health departments with their district offices, and the various divisions of the United States Department of Health, Education and Welfare (HEW). All employ health educators in various capacities in order to reach the public with their health messages.

Most of the state and national professional organizations employ health educators to make the public aware of certain health problems and their solutions. Professional associations are groups of individuals with a common background of service, a systematic curriculum and training, and some form of certification which legally allows them to practice their profession. Among the professional organizations employing health educators are the American Medical Association, the American Dental Association, and the American Association of Health, Physical Education and Recreation.

STUDENT PROJECTS

1. Poll a number of other students who are not members of this class to determine what types of health services were available to them in elementary and secondary school.
2. Report on the environmental factors in your present surroundings which have a direct impact on either the mental or the physical health of students.

GLOSSARY OF TERMS

Health   That quality of life which permits an individual to function to an optimal degree within his environment.

School health education   All the activities of the school and its environment which have an impact on the health of students and all other school personnel.

Health instruction   Dissemination of health knowledge in order to develop concepts concerning specific health problems and to ensure good health practices.

Health services   Those activities which appraise, conserve, and protect the health of the student.

Healthful school environment   Physical and other conditions in the school which are conducive to the promotion of good health practices.

REFERENCES

1. Cyrus Mayshark and Leslie W. Irwin, *Health Education in Secondary Schools,* 3d ed. (St. Louis: C. V. Mosby, 1972), p. 33.

SELECTED READINGS

Anderson, C. L. *Community Health.* St. Louis: C. V. Mosby, 1973.

Anderson, C. L., and Creswell, William H. Jr. *School Health Practice.* 6th ed. St. Louis: C. V. Mosby, 1973.

Bucher, Charles A.; Olsen, Einar A.; and Willgoose, Carl E. *The Foundations of Health.* 2d ed. Englewood Cliffs, N.J.: Prentice-Hall, 1976.

Byrd, Oliver E. *School Health Administration.* Philadelphia: W. B. Saunders, 1964.

Haag, Jessie Helen. *School Health Program.* Rev. ed. New York: Holt, Rinehart and Winston, 1967.

Jenne, Frank H., and Greene, Walter H. *Turner's School Health and Health Education.* 7th ed. St. Louis: C. V. Mosby, 1976.

Mayshark, Cyrus, and Irwin, Leslie W. *Health Education in Secondary Schools.* 3d ed. St. Louis: C. V. Mosby, 1972.

Mayshark, Cyrus, and Shaw, Donald. *Administration of School Health Programs.* St. Louis: C. V. Mosby, 1967.

Osborn, Barbara M.; Means, Richard K.; Smolensky, Jack; and Sawrey, James M. *Foundation of Health Sciences.* Boston: Allyn and Bacon, 1968.

Means, Richard K. *A History of Health Education in the United States.* Philadelphia: Lea & Febiger, 1963.

Nemir, Alma. *The School Health Program.* Philadelphia: W. B. Saunders, 1970.

Oberteuffer, Delbert, and Beyrer, Mary K. *School Health Education.* 4th ed. New York: Harper & Row, 1966.

Stiles, William W. *Individual and Community Health.* New York: McGraw-Hill, 1953.

Chapter 13
The Profession's Responsibilities for Adult Fitness

Health and fitness are not the province solely of the young.

ANONYMOUS

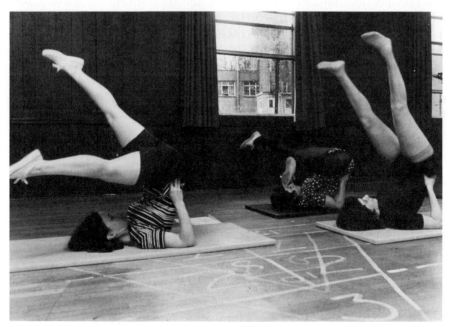

Classes in "slimnastics" are popular with adult women.

THE TWO great wars in our immediate past (World War I, 1917–1918, and World War II, 1941–1945) served to bring to the attention of the American public the lack of physical fitness of its citizens, especially the adult male. Sixteen and 33 percent respectively of the potential inductees were rejected for military service in these wars. In the aftermath of both wars changes were made to raise the level of fitness in what should have been the healthiest segment of the population. After World War I, twenty-one states adopted mandatory physical education in the schools. After World War II a Council on Youth Fitness was appointed by the President as a result of the high rejection rates in World War II and the results of the Kraus-Weber tests which showed that American children compared poorly with European children on the same test. Over twenty years have transpired since this latter event and, although some progress has been made, the problem of adult fitness is still with us. The conflicts in Korea and Vietnam involved relatively few soldiers, sailors, and marines from the available manpower pool. The rejection rates therefore were meaningless since only the most fit were retained.

Many people, both within and outside of the professions of physical education and medicine, have reported all types of benefits to be derived from exercise for adults. Some of the more outlandish claims have done more harm than good since the intelligent and/or skeptical adult wishes substantiation for such claims. If none is forthcoming, the value of exercise remains questionable. Conversely, when sophisticated research studies support the benefits that can accrue from good exercise programs, such programs gain adult acceptance.

A number of reliable studies have been conducted concerning the effect of prolonged exercise on the human physiology. Some of these studies have indicated the role of exercise in preventive medicine. One such study is the ten-year study reported by Golding. In summarizing the effects of exercise on the subjects he states:

> The original cholesterol levels were slightly high possibly because the subjects were primarily upper-socio-economic; white collar; sedentary workers. During the first year there was a significant reduction in serum cholesterol. This trend continued in the second year and third year. During the fourth and fifth years the cholesterol level increased. It plateaued in the sixth year and although it had increased considerably it was still significantly below the original levels. A secondary reduction occurred in the seventh year which coincided with the national interest in jogging, and we added more running to the program.
>
> Skinfold fat measurements displayed a pattern similar to that of cholesterol. After being reduced for the first two years, it increased and leveled off at a value well below the original measurement.

Weight has not changed during a ten-year period. Subjects remained the same weight which emphasizes the fact that weight is sometimes a misleading measurement. A scale is just measuring mass, and does not give body composition. A boy weighing 200 lbs. and who is six feet tall could be simply obese if much of the weight is fat, or could be an athlete if the weight was muscle. Weight in itself is not as important as the body composition. In our study weight did not change but fat was reduced, reflecting a change in body composition. Subjects lost fat but gained muscle density.

Physical Working Capacity also improved significantly; it is usually believed that as a man gets older there is a drastic reduction in his working capacity. Our data contradicts this belief. A few years ago while testing incoming freshmen at Kent State University we observed that the men in the experimental exercise program with a mean age of 47 years outperformed incoming freshmen with an average age of 18. Resting heart rate, recovery heart rate, and their ability to transport oxygen, all have shown significant improvement although after initial gains, many have plateaued. These men are eleven years older and they are resisting a normal aging trend. If a subject actually stayed the same over the ten years, it would be desirable because he would be preventing the normal decrease in fitness due to age. These subjects actually reversed the aging trend in most measures.[1]

Despite such findings, the public is bombarded by advertisements of "get-fit-quick" programs conducted in spas and recommended by sports figures and entertainers, or offered home programs which use some ingenious device which takes the work out of becoming fit. Both provide the risk of a loss of money, no results, and possible physical injury. This latter statement does not include the "health clubs" which may be run by professionally competent personnel and under the supervision of proper medical personnel.

Physical fitness may be attained at home, at clubs, at recreational facilities, or at educational institutions. One becomes aware of this by observing the activities of adults most any evening or weekend. Golf, walking, tennis, and jogging are examples of activities which provide the populace with varying levels of fitness opportunities. Some of these activities and programs will be explained in ensuing paragraphs.

Unfortunately, in the past, schools and colleges assumed that if the student were provided with a "gym" program in school that (a) its responsibilities were complete and (b) the students would continue to perform physical activities in the future. It seems that both assumptions were in error. The profession of physical education has a responsibility for adult fitness and many so-called "gym" programs were so poor that not only did the adult cease to perform physical activities after leaving school but he or she was left with a feeling of revulsion toward physical education and fitness programs. As a result, a schism developed between school physical education and the adult who needed to be fit in order to function more readily, enjoy recreational activities, and enjoy life to a greater degree. To fill this void several programs, as sponsored by individuals or agencies, came into being. Some of these are headed by professional physical educators, others by medical personnel. More recently the two have blended to provide programs in the area of adult fitness and the necessary research to advance it.

One of the more accepted programs of fitness which can be conducted on an individual basis is the aerobics program espoused by Cooper. This program is based upon a variety of exercises which stimulate the cardiovascular system and produce beneficial changes. Examples of these exercises are swimming and running. The objective of the program is to increase the amount of oxygen that the body can utilize in a given time. The concept of Cooper's program is that the more vigorous the activity the less of it one must do to get or maintain fitness. His point system is based on the caloric cost of activity. The program is geared to all age levels and the fitness of the individuals within those levels. The starter program in each age level determines the time, distance, and frequency of the walking and running aspects of the program. All are predicated on the premise that the participant has had a good physical examination preceding entrance to the program.

Individual jogging programs have been the subject of much publicity, both good and bad. Unfortunately, the news media have reported a number of incidents in which joggers have had heart attacks while jogging resulting, in some cases, in death. Such misfortunes, however, are still rare enough to be news; hundreds of individuals die each night

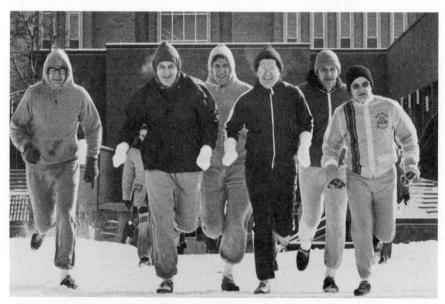

Jogging is a popular medium through which physical fitness can be achieved. Photo courtesy of Exercise Physiology Laboratory, Kent State University.

in bed. In many cases, the jogger was an unconditioned person, had not had a physical examination, and had an unknown cardiac deficiency. Jogging, properly conducted, is probably the fastest growing activity in America. Its benefits are great, the equipment and facilities needed are minimal, and it can be geared to include all members of the family. The precaution of a physical examination should be mandatory for anyone over the age of 35 embarking on such a program.

No other agency or institution has contributed so much to the area of physical fitness as the YMCA. Its program, as explained in its publication *The Y's Way to Physical Fitness,* is an outstanding example of this service to the adult. In addition to its organizational contributions, the chapters on fitness testing and exercise programs merit serious study and consideration. The YMCA constantly upgrades both its programs and its personnel by a series of workshops and seminars.

In recent years cardiologists have become concerned that a number of persons, especially in upper age brackets engage in physical activities without proper conditioning and at times with physical deficiencies which may endanger their lives. Even a normal physical examination may not reveal some cardiac problems which may appear under stress. As an answer to this problem, a number of exercise physiologists and cardiologists have devised a system of exercise stress testing in which the would-be participant is stressed by increasing exercise to determine at what point there may be a gap between myocardial oxygen supply and demand. The usual practice involves the use of a bicycle ergometer or treadmill and the subject or patient. The subject is carefully monitored during the test. ECG tracings are recorded as the work load is gradually increased and any abnormality usually ends the test. An exercise program is then prescribed for the subject which is within the limits of the test results; it may vary from a single walking program to a vigorous game of handball. The medical profession is also using this program to determine the activity level of patients who are referred to them. This program, still in its infancy, should be of great benefit as more and more research data becomes available.

The profession of physical education must assume its share of responsibility for the physical condition of adults. The average life expectancy for all born in the United States is now more than seventy years. There is an increasing need for improved fitness programs for those adults who are not in a position to pay for the opportunity to keep fit or are not located in those areas where facilities are available. Members of the profession will find employment in agencies outside the educational sphere. In states where older citizens retire, such employment may be in programs for the aged.

STUDENT PROJECTS

1. Have reports on adult fitness programs available to all college or university personnel—both academic and nonacademic.

2. Have students describe adult fitness programs or opportunities available in their home towns or cities.

GLOSSARY OF TERMS

Cholesterol   A steroid alcohol found in animal cells and body fluids and a factor in arteriosclerosis.

Stress testing   Testing by means of subjecting testee to graduated exercise under close supervision.

Treadmill   An apparatus to test walking or running capacity by use of a driven tread and an adjustable incline plane.

Bicycle ergometer   Bicycle with adjustable resistance and device for measuring the amount of work done.

REFERENCES

1. Lawrence A. Golding, "Cholesterol and Exercise," *YMCA Journal of Physical Education* (March–April 1972), pp. 106–110. Reprinted by permission.

SELECTED READINGS

American College of Sports Medicine. *Guidelines for Graded Exercise Testing and Exercise Prescription.* Philadelphia: Lea & Febiger, 1975.

Clarke, David H., *Exercise Physiology.* Englewood Cliffs, N.J.: Prentice-Hall, 1975.

Cooper, Kenneth H. *The New Aerobics.* New York: Bantam Books, 1970.

Cureton, Thomas Kirk. *The Physiological Effects of Exercise Programs on Adults.* Springfield, Ill.: Charles C Thomas, 1969.

Myers, Clayton R. *The Official YMCA Physical Fitness Handbook.* New York: Popular Library, 1975.

The Y's Way to Physical Fitness. National Council, YMCA, U.S.A., 1973.

Wilson, Philip K. *Adult Fitness and Cardiac Rehabilitation.* Baltimore: University Park Press, 1975.

YMCA, "Special Report National YMCA Physical Fitness Consultation." *Journal of Physical Education* (March–April 1972).

Chapter 14
Responsibilities as a Member of a Profession

In time a profession is like marriage, we cease to note anything but its inconveniences.

BALZAC

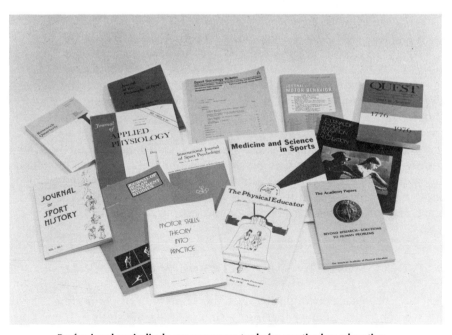

Professional periodicals are necessary tools for continuing education.

A PROFESSION utilizes the application of knowledge acquired through the study of a discipline. Because the term "profession" is misused to include many nonprofessional areas, it can be confusing. How does one distinguish between those positions which are professional and those which are not? What are the characteristics of a profession?

Characteristics of a Profession

The nature of a profession differs from that of a trade, a business, or entertainment. The fact that one does or does not get paid for doing work has little to do with the professional nature of the work. One of the better lists of criteria of a profession, distributed as a memo by the Ohio Commission for Teacher Education, follows.

1. A profession involves activities essentially intellectual.
2. A profession commands a body of specialized knowledge.
3. A profession requires extended professional (as contrasted with solely general) preparation.
4. A profession demands continuous in-service growth.
5. A profession affords a life career and permanent membership.
6. A profession sets up its own standards.
7. A profession exalts service above personal gain.
8. A profession has a strong, closely knit, professional organization.
9. A profession enters into a covenant with its clientele.[1]

One does not become a member of a profession merely by signing a contract for money, as does the baseball or football professional athlete. One becomes a professional through a series of preparatory steps which are discussed in the following paragraphs.

A profession develops when there is a sufficient, unique body of knowledge to support its membership. This definition does not preclude the derivation of background information from other disciplines, but it does imply an accumulation of knowledge about one subject which is not common to other disciplines or professions.

A STUDENT MOVES TOWARD BECOMING A PROFESSIONAL

Teaching physical education involves the same type of commitment and involvement as does any other profession. Among the steps in becoming a professional are the following.

1. *Selecting a university or college with a good course of study in the field of choice.* This first step involves those students who are attending junior colleges or two-year community colleges as well as those who are selecting a four-year institution. The course of study should involve general courses in the liberal arts, specific courses in education, and courses in the major field. No college or university can give the student experiences in all the physical activities he or she may be expected to teach or coach. Universities usually offer those most often taught in that particular locale. Additional skills are acquired at clinics, conventions, and in-service workshops. The new teacher is not expected to be an expert in all sports activities. The ability to teach and analyze is much more important.

Deficiencies in the physical-activities background of prospective teachers can be removed, but the time spent in this removal could better be spent in other facets of professional preparation. In addition, if the university of college has a high set of professional standards, that fact increases the possibilities for employment and acceptance for future graduate studies.

2. *Beginning a professional library.* The major student should begin to acquire a personal, professional library with his or her first courses in school. Unlike the lawyer and the doctor, whose initial libraries may be an expensive venture, the professional physical educator may obtain an adequate library at modest cost. Nevertheless, he or she may become the resource person in the community on activity buildings and the dimensions of playing areas for sports. Books from early courses serve as reference materials for later ones. Books should be supplemented by professional journals as soon as possible to ensure a source of current research and literature.

In addition to beginning a personal library, the professional student must learn to use the research facilities available in modern college and university libraries. The interlibrary loan policy opens up unlimited resources. Proper use of the library is basic to one's professional growth.

3. *Joining professional student major clubs.* Most teacher-education institutions have professional and sports interest clubs. The former have the advantage of fostering professional growth among the members. Two national fraternities (Delta Psi Kappa for women, and Phi Epsilon Kappa for men) have chartered units on many campuses. Interest clubs give the students an opportunity to improve their skills in activities which may have limited exposure in the curriculum.

4. *Joining professional organizations.* Most of the state associations have special student membership dues, sections in periodicals, and student sections at conventions. Students elect their own officers and are represented on the representative assembly or its equivalent.

Recently the American Association for Health, Physical Education and Recreation announced the appointment of two staff consultants who are to assume the responsibilities of coordinating the student section and major club development. The district conventions of AAHPER and the national convention have placement services available to help the members, including students.

5. *Attending workshops and clinics.* Since the curriculum cannot include all the activities in various programs, and since many of those offered cannot be covered in depth, most universities, colleges, and sports associations offer a number of workshops, clinics, and institutes. Usually the speakers are nationally known educators, players, and coaches. The student may never again have access to so many talented professionals. Some workshops, especially those of several weeks' duration, carry academic credit.

6. *Attaining the highest academic achievement.* Since there is no such thing as terminal education, and since most states certify the beginning teacher only provisionally, additional schooling beyond the baccalaureate degree will be necessary. It is advantageous to maintain grades above average in order to gain admission to graduate studies rather than continue work on the undergraduate level. The work taken toward permanent certification can then apply to an advanced degree. A good academic average ensures the student a choice of schools and levels he or she wishes to pursue.

CONTINUED PROFESSIONAL GROWTH

Any profession depends on its membership for the leadership that commands the respect of other fields of study. Such men as Sargent, Hetherington, Wood, Williams, Nash, and others have brought the profession up a long hard road. The present leadership has continued to follow the examples of these great men. The leadership of the future will be provided by the present group of students and young teachers who must prepare themselves for the future. Such preparation includes the following:

1. *Membership in professional organizations.* The American Alliance for Health, Physical Education and Recreation, the American College of Sports Medicine, the American School Health Association, the National Association of Physical Education for College Women, the National College Physical Education Association for Men, and the National Recreation and Park Association are among the organizations available to the organizations available to the professional physical educator. These organizations develop and disseminate new ideas in the field, offer consultative services to the membership, provide opportunities (through

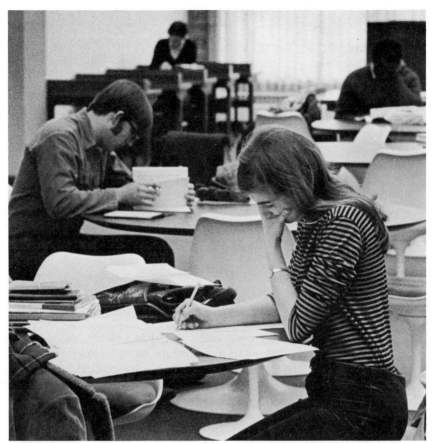

In addition to establishing their own libraries, students should use existing library facilities. Photo courtesy of Kent State University News Service.

journals and meetings) for debating and discussing vital issues, and serve as a medium for employment information. Recently, the national organizations have become more active politically in areas that concern their members. In order to upgrade the areas of health, physical education, and recreation, workers in those fields should join professional associations as most members of the legal or medical profession do.

2. *Advanced study.* Work beyond the baccalaureate degree is required by most states for a life or permanent certificate. This work may be a continuation of meaningful undergraduate work or study toward an advanced degree. Since most school systems relate salary range to degree attainments, study beyond the baccalaureate is best spent working toward an advanced degree.

The teacher should exert the same care and planning in selecting a graduate school that he or she exercised in selecting an undergraduate school. Unfortunately, the choice of graduate schools may be limited by the teacher's performance at the undergraduate level. In a 1967 study, Resick found that 103 of 151 institutions required at least a C+ average for admission.[2] Other factors considered were a major or minor in the field, a specific average for the final two years, letters of recommendation, and a standard entrance examination. Some of the institutions surveyed accepted graduate students on probation when their qualifications were slightly below the acceptable standards. Thus there are strong reasons for the stress on good academic achievement at the undergraduate level.

3. *Attendance at conventions, workshops, clinics, and in-service meetings.* The athletic coaches in their specialties take this means to growth more seriously than do other teachers. Failing to keep up with new ideas in athletics helps to ensure an early professional demise. Teachers in the classroom, in the gymnasiums, or on the playing fields are not reviewed by the public every week, and they may tend to become complacent. That one belongs to a professional organization is not enough; new ideas come from reading the research and ideas expressed in the journals. New ideas also come from exchanges at conventions, including informal ones in the elevators and the lobbies of hotels. The authors consider a convention successful if it has uncovered one hot, usable idea, and the same criterion can be applied to a workshop or clinic. Better methods, newer approaches and a better insight into problems usually result from such attendance.[3] Conventions cover a variety of areas within a field. Clinics ordinarily cover one sport or activity. Workshops center on a specific area within a field of study. Finally, in-service meetings are based on the needs of the group. All have one goal in common—to upgrade the teachers in a school system or within a discipline.

4. *Research and writing.* The life blood of any profession is its growth and development through philosophic concepts and ideas expressed in its professional journals and research reported in its research publications. A discipline exists only if it has a unique body of knowledge. Ideas may be lost if they are not recorded and disseminated to the membership. A profession that merely maintains the status quo stagnates.

New methods, new activities, means of evaluation and its effect on people—these are the results of research. Although no professional likes to be faced with the old threat of "publish or perish," many professionals need to be prodded off "dead center." By demanding an investigation of what now exists, research in itself improves the individual. In describing the reasons for research, Steinhaus answered the question "Why this research?" by resort to analogy:

> Woodchopping produces both useful wood and a better woodchopper. Research must give to our fields the building materials of accurate facts and principles with which to construct sound practice

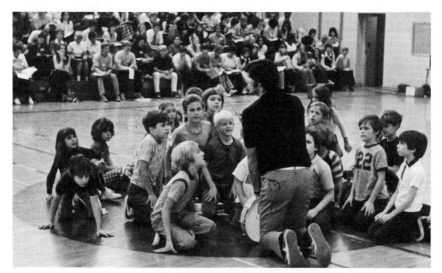

Attendance at workshops is one method of continued professional growth. Photo courtesy of Department of Physical Education, Kent State University.

and wise philosophy. It must supply ideas to kindle enthusiasm in our professional ranks and, in the public mind, a warm reception for our programs.[4]

5. *Excellence in teaching.* The professional approaches each day, each class, and each assignment with the hope of doing the best possible job. Good teaching is the base of any teaching field. Every lesson should be evaluated as to its effect on the plans for the course. Every teacher's class receives an evaluation from the students as they leave. It may be a simple comment such as "a waste of time" or "enjoyable lesson" or "good class."

In some institutions rewards tend to be given mostly to those who are involved in research or writing, since these two facets of teaching are easy to measure. In the past several years a real effort has been made to identify those individuals who excel in the classroom and to give them monetary awards, plaques, or simply titles like "teacher of the year."

As the educator becomes more professional, he or she becomes aware of the broader aspects of the field and of all education.

Each educator has a five-way concern in his educative efforts. By no priority but by a sequence of logic it might be stated that the first concern is for the *student.* The second concern is for the *subject matter.* The third concern is for the *profession of specialization.* The fourth concern is for the *total education enterprise,* and the fifth concern is toward *man in the world.* The good teacher may find only the first two ways to be concerned—for the student and for his own subject matter. The true professional concerns himself with the first, the second, the third, the fourth, and the fifth educational endeavors.[5]

RESPONSIBILITIES AS A PROFESSIONAL

In addition to performing their duties in a professional manner, professionals have several other responsibilities. By their work, research, speeches, and writing they contribute to the advancement of their profession.

A true professional in physical education is interested and informed about the other disciplines within the school. He or she is knowledgeable in the area of philosophy of education being pursued within the school system and the contributions of his or her field toward the objectives of the school. The professional also interprets this field to his or her colleagues and to the community in order that others may understand the program and its accomplishments and, in turn, develops interest in community projects and assists others in pursuing them. Professionals in all fields serve the community in many leadership roles.

THE FUTURE OF THE PROFESSION

Since World War II, physical education in the United States has enjoyed greater status than at any other time in its history. Because of the poor physical condition of many Selective Service inductees and later because of the inferiority of American children to their European counterparts in physical fitness, the nation became aware of a growing problem. President Eisenhower formed a President's Council of Fitness to bring to the attention of all the problem of an unfit citizenry. Throughout the nation, the press gave more favorable coverage than ever before to the activities of those involved in bringing the physical fitness message to the people.

Recent evidence points to a beneficial effect of physical fitness on longevity and especially cardiovascular health. The shortening of the workweek and the continuation of a trend toward complete mechanization suggest the need for good physical education in the future. And finally, the need for some new forms of physical activity for those who will spend long periods of time in space adds another dimension to the program in the future. A field of endeavor that has survived several thousand years will continue to flourish in spite of the competition for the school time and the tax dollar.

CAREER OPPORTUNITIES IN PHYSICAL EDUCATION

A student who graduates from a good undergraduate or graduate program has many job opportunities in physical education and related fields. The principal ones are the teaching and coaching positions at all educational levels. In compliance with Title IX, the opportunities for coaching, athletic training, and athletic administration for women have increased immeasurably. At the higher levels of education there is generally a need for specialization in some area of the discipline in addition to a good pedagogical background. Examples of such specializations include aquatics, athletic training, athletic administration, dance, elementary school physical education, the history and philosophy of physical education, motor behavior, physiology of exercise, biomechanics, and adaptive physical education.

An increasing number of job opportunities are available in related fields as well. Such opportunities can be divided into the following categories:

1. Commercial—opportunities in health clubs, tourist groups, and professional sports.
2. Educational—sports administration, athletic training, and physical education for exceptional children.
3. Public and Service Organizations—Physical instructors in YMCA-YWCA, instructors in fitness programs for the aged, and physical education instructors in rehabilitative institutions.

CONCLUSIONS

People do not become professionals overnight. Most of the burden to instill a professional attitude remains with the teacher-education institution and the major department. If students are taught by professors who do not keep up to date, who lack a professional attitude, who do not conduct research or write, and who themselves are not members of professional associations, there is little chance that the students will develop a professional attitude. If the students have no contact with professional growth opportunities during their undergraduate days, there is little likelihood that they will seek them out later. The major department has an obligation that goes far beyond the offerings of courses which satisfy the state's minimum certification requirements.

STUDENT PROJECTS

1. List the ten characteristics you most admire in teachers you have had at all levels of instruction.
2. Review graduate school bulletins to compare academic requirements for admission.
3. Present summaries of the leading professional organizations, especially those open to students.

GLOSSARY OF TERMS

Profession An occupation requiring specialized knowledge, guided by principles, and involving long and intensive academic preparation.

Workshop   A seminar emphasizing free discussion and participation by all members.

Institute   A short series of meetings on a specic subject.

Clinic   A series of meetings on a specific physical activity for the purpose of updating the practitioners.

REFERENCES

1. Ohio Commission on Teacher Education and Professional Standards. *TEPS and the Teaching Profession: A Position Statement and Concerns.* Memorandum to local Teachers Associations, Columbus, May 22, 1969.
2. Matthew C. Resick, "Graduate Patterns," address presented at the Graduate Education Conference, Washington, January 8, 1967.
3. Matthew C. Resick, "Let's Turn Pro," *The Physical Educator* **17** (December 1960), pp. 135–136.
4. Arthur H. Steinhaus, "Why This Research?" in *Research Methods,* 2d ed, ed. M. G. Scott (Washington: American Association for Health, Physical Education and Recreation, 1959), p. 17.
5. Leona Holbrook, "Education Is Our Business," *Journal of Health, Physical Education and Recreation* **37** (April 1966), pp. 19, 81.

SELECTED READINGS

Angell, George. "Physical Education and the New Breed." *Journal of Health, Physical Education and Recreation* **40** (June 1969), pp. 25–28.

Bookwalter, Carolyn, and Bookwalter, Karl. "How Professional Is Physical Education?" *The Foil* (Spring 1975), pp. 34–41.

Holbrook, Leona. "Education Is Our Business." *Journal of Health, Physical Education and Recreation* **37** (April 1966), pp. 19, 81.

NAPECW-NCPEAM *Careers in Physical Education.* Washington, D.C.: AAHPER, 1975.

Nixon, John E., and Jewett, Ann E. *An Introduction to Physical Education.* 7th ed. Philadelphia: W. B. Saunders, 1969.

Ohio Commission on Teaching Education and Professional Standards. *TEPS and the Teaching Profession: A Position Statement and Concerns.* Memorandum to local Teachers Associations. Columbus, Ohio, May 22, 1969.

Resick, Matthew C. "Graduate Patterns." Speech presented at the Graduate Education Conference, Washington, January 8, 1967.

————. "Let's Turn Pro." *The Physical Educator* **17** (December 1960), pp. 135–36.

Scott, M. Gladys, ed. *Research Methods.* 2d ed. Washington: American Association for Health, Physical Education and Recreation, 1959.

Singer, Robert N., ed. *Physical Education: Foundations.* New York: Holt, Rinehart and Winston, 1976.

Index